Asger Frandsen, Public Health Aspects of Periodontal Disease

Public Health Aspects of Periodontal Disease

Proceedings of a workshop held in Copenhagen, Denmark
December 3–5, 1982

Sponsored by the Commission of the European Communities,
as advised by the Committee on Medical and Public
Health Research

Edited by

Asger Frandsen

Royal Dental College
Copenhagen, Denmark

Quintessence Publishing Co., Inc.   1984
Chicago, London, Berlin, Rio de Janeiro and Tokyo

© 1984 by ECSC, EEC, EAEC, Brussels and Luxembourg
Published by Quintessence Publishing Co., Inc., Chicago for
Commission of the European Communities,
Directorate-General Information Market
and Innovation, Luxembourg

EUR 8960

Composition and printing: Ernst Kieser GmbH, Augsburg
Binding: Lüderitz & Bauer-GmbH, Berlin
Printed in Germany
ISBN 0-86715-153-6

Preface

This book contains the proceedings of a workshop on 'Public Health Aspects of Periodontal Disease' held in Copenhagen, Denmark, December 3–5, 1982.

The workshop was a follow-up of a previous workshop held in Dublin, Ireland, December 12–14, 1979, with the title *Efficacy of Treatment Procedures in Periodontics*, and from which the proceedings were published in 1980.

The general purpose of the present workshop was to analyze the problem which periodontal disease constitutes in the European Community and to suggest ways in which this problem may be alleviated. Objectives under this purpose were:

1. Identification of problem.
2. Analysis of existing dental care delivery services.
3. Goal formulations, strategies and manpower.

Participants mainly representing the member states of the European Community were invited to the workshop, together with representatives from Finland, Sweden and Switzerland. Seventeen workpapers pertaining to the subjects of the workshop were prepared by some of the participants and distributed prior to the meeting. It was not intended that these papers should be read at the meeting, but rather that they should form the background for group and plenum discussions which constituted the main activity of the workshop.

The workpapers, together with summaries of group and plenum discussions, are presented in this book.

Acknowledgements

The workshop was held under the auspices of the European Commission and was recommended by its Committee for Medical and Public Health Research (CRM). Travel costs, lodging and meals, meeting facilities as well as other activities involved in the conduct of the workshop and the preparation of the proceedings were paid for by the Commission.

The official Danish delegate to the CRMs 'Specialized Working Group on Medical Biology', Professor *Mogens Hauge,* University of Odense, and the Chairman of the CRM, Professor *Bent Sørensen,* Hvidovre Hospital, Copenhagen, were active in the developing of the project through the EEC channels. Dr *Emilio Levi,* secretary to the 'Specialized Working Group' has given valuable advice prior to, during and after the workshop concerning all organizational matters.

The Danish Dental Association kindly accepted to house the workshop and also held a reception for the participants.

Pia Jørgensen, Lise Svendsen and *Ulla Jacobsen* performed efficiently as secretaries during the meeting, and *Ulla Jacobsen* has been most helpful in the organization of the workshop and the preparation of the proceedings. The British and the Irish participants rendered valuable assistance by performing language correction of the manuscripts prepared by authors not having English as their mother tongue.

The nucleus of a workshop, like the present, comprises the workpapers and the competence − in diverse areas − of the participants. The seriousness with which all participants took part in the deliberations made this workshop a success.

List of Participants

Professor Jukka Ainamo
Department of Periodontology
Institute of Dentistry
University of Helsinki
Mannerheimintie 172
SF-00280 Helsinki 28
Finland

Professor Rolf Attström
Department of Periodontology
Dental School
Carl Gustavsväg 34
S 214 21 Malmö
Sweden

Dr David E. Barmes
Chief, Oral Health
World Health Organization
1211 Geneva 27
Switzerland

Professor Axel Bergenholtz
Department of Periodontology
School of Dentistry
University of Umeå
S 901 87 Umeå
Sweden

Dr Jan De Boever
Department of Fixed Prosthesis and
Periodontology
Academic Hospital
De Pintelaan 185
B-9000 Gent
Belgium

Dr Gert Borring-Møller
Tårnvej 219
DK-2610 Rødovre
Denmark

Dr Noel M. Claffey
University of Dublin
Dental School
Trinity College
Dublin 2
Ireland

Dr John J. Clarkson
Act. Chief Dental Officer
Department of Health, Room 419
Hawkins House
Dublin 2
Ireland

Dr Michael H. Craft
Director of the HEC Dental Health Study
University of Cambridge
Addenbrooke's Hospital
Trumpington Street
GB-Cambridge CB2 1QE
United Kingdom

Dr Martin C. Downer
Chief Dental Officer
Scottish Home and Health Department
Saint Andrew's House
Regent Road
Edinburgh EH1 3DE
United Kingdom

Professor Lavinia Flores-de-Jacoby
Department of Periodontology
Medicine School of Dentistry
Philipps University
Georg-Voigt-Str. 3
D-3550 Marburg
West Germany

Professor Asger Frandsen
Department of Periodontology
Royal Dental College
Jagtvej 160
DK-2100 Copenhagen Ø
Denmark

Professor Mogens Hauge
University Institute of Clinical Genetics
Odense Hospital
J. B. Winsløws Vej 17
DK-5000 Odense C
Denmark

Professor Sven Helm
Institute for Community Dentistry and
Postgraduate Studies
Royal Dental College
Jagtvej 155.B
DK-2200 Copenhagen N
Denmark

Dr Jos L. M. van den Heuvel
Consultant, Ziekenfondsraad
Prof. J. H. Bavincklaan 2
NL-1183 AT Amstelveen
The Netherlands

Dr Robert Jacoby
Bahnhofstrasse 13
D-3550 Marburg
West Germany

Associate Professor Thorkild Karring
Department of Periodontology
Royal Dental College
Vennelyst Boulevard
DK-8000 Århus C
Denmark

Professor Arnd F. Käyser
Catholic University
Department of Occlusal Reconstruction
Philips van Leydenlaan 25
NL-6500 HB Nijmegen
The Netherlands

Professor Jacques Kohl
Institut de Stomatologie
Hôpital de Bavière
B-4020 Liège
Belgium

Dr Henri S. Koskas
Editor: *Journal de Parodontologie*
43, Rue des Petits Champs
F-75001 Paris
France

Professor Wolfgang Krüger
Department of Operative Dentistry
and Periodontology
Dental School
University of Göttingen
Robert-Koch-Str. 40
D-3400 Göttingen
West Germany

Professor Klaus G. König
University of Nijmegen
Faculty of Medicine and Dentistry
NL-Nijmegen
The Netherlands

Professor Niklaus P. Lang
University of Berne
School of Dental Medicine
Freiburgstr. 7
CH-3010 Berne
Switzerland

Professor Dieter E. Lange
Department of Periodontics
University of Münster
Waldeyer Str. 30
D-4400 Münster
West Germany

Dr Jørgen Langebæk
Danish Dental Association
Amaliegade 17
DK-1256 Copenhagen K
Denmark

Mr Michael A. Lennon
Department of Child Dental Health
University Dental Hospital of Manchester
Bridgeford Street
Manchester M15 6FH
United Kingdom

Dr Emilio Levi
Biology Division D. G. XII
CEC
Centro Commune di Ricerca
I-21020 Ispra
Italy

Professor Thomas Marthaler
Department of Oral Epidemiology
and Preventive Dentistry
Dental Institute
Postfach 8028
CH-Zurich
Switzerland

Professor Jean Martin
Université de Nancy 1
Groupe INSERM U.115
Facultés de Médecine
Avenue de la Forêt de Haye
B.P.184-54000 Vandoeuvre-lès-Nancy
France

Dr Ingolf Møller
Regional Officer for Oral Health
World Health Organization
Scherfigsvej 8
DK-2100 Copenhagen Ø
Denmark

Professor Taco Pilot
Faculty of Odontology
University of Groningen
Ant. Deusinglaan 1
NL-9713 AV Groningen
The Netherlands

Chief Dental Officer Eli Schwarz
National Board of Health
Store Kongensgade 1
DK-1264 Copenhagen K
Denmark

Dr Diarmuid B. Shanley
Director of Dental School
University of Dublin
Dental School
Trinity College
Dublin 2
Ireland

Dr Aubrey Sheiham
The London Hospital Medical College
University of London
Dental School
Turner Street
London E1 2AD
United Kingdom

Associate Professor Mogens R.
Skougaard
Institute for Community Dentistry
and Postgraduate Studies
Royal Dental College
Jagtvej 155.B
DK-2200 Copenhagen N
Denmark

Professor Daniel van Steenberghe
Department of Periodontology
School of Dentistry, Oral Pathology
and Oral Surgery, Faculty of Medicine
Catholic University of Leuven
Kapucijnenvoer 7
B-3000 Leuven
Belgium

Associate Professor Kaj Stoltze
Department of Periodontology
Royal Dental College
Jagtvej 160
DK-2100 Copenhagen Ø
Denmark

9

Dr Göran Söderholm
Dental Care Clinic
Kockums AB
Box 832
S 201 80 Malmö
Sweden

Professor Bent Sørensen
Department of Plastic Surgery
and Burns Unit
Hvidovre Hospital
Kettegaard Alle 30
DK-2650 Hvidovre
Denmark

Dr Poul Thorpen Teglers
School of Dental Hygienists and
Chairside Assistants
Royal Dental College

Møllegade 25
DK-2200 Copenhagen N
Denmark

Associate Professor Jørgen Theilade
Department of Electron Microscopy
Royal Dental College
Vennelyst Boulevard
DK-8000 Århus C
Denmark

Dr Giorgio Vogel
Chairman, Department of Stomatology
Medical Faculty, University of Milano
Instituto di Scienze Biomediche
St. Paolo
Via Di Rudini 8
I-20142 Milano
Italy

Organizing Committee

Professor Asger Frandsen, (Chairman and Editor) Royal Dental College, Copenhagen

Dr Jørgen Langebæk, Danish Dental Association, Copenhagen

Dr Ingolf Møller, Regional Officer for Oral Health, WHO, Copenhagen

Associate Professor Mogens R. Skougaard, Royal Dental College, Copenhagen

Dr Poul Thorpen Teglers, Royal Dental College, Copenhagen

Honorary Members

Chairman of the EEC 'Comité de Recherche Médicale' Professor Bent Sørensen, Hvidovre Hospital, Copenhagen

Danish Delegate to the EEC 'Specialized Working Group on Medical Biology' Professor Mogens Hauge, Odense University Hospital, Odense

President of the Danish Dental Association Dr Bent Skaanild, Danish Dental Association, Copenhagen

Secretariat

Associate Professor Kaj Stoltze, Royal Dental College, Copenhagen

Ulla Jacobsen, Royal Dental College, Copenhagen

Pia Jørgensen, Danish Dental Association, Copenhagen

Lise Svendsen, Royal Dental College, Copenhagen

Introduction

For a long time destructive periodontal disease has been recognized as a major oral disorder. The problem derives its magnitude from the fact that almost all adult people all over the world suffer from some degree of the disease and that it is considered responsible for a substantial part of the tooth loss. Further, whereas its aetiology is fairly well clarified, and effective preventive and therapeutic measures have been demonstrated in human model systems, population control of the disease has not yet been realized.

In December 1979 a workshop, under the auspices of the European Commission, was convened in Dublin, Ireland, to consider the efficacy of periodontal treatment. The main emphasis was on the application of periodontal treatment on a community basis in Europe. One recommendation from the proceedings of that workshop reads: 'The organization of further Workshops for the initiation/concerted action to collate existing knowledge in all aspects of periodontal disease'.

The present workshop was particularly aimed at Public Health problems related to periodontal disease and periodontal care in the member states of the European Community.

These aspects comprise the prevalence, the health consequences, and the socioeconomic impact of periodontal disease, and large scale measures for prevention and treatment of periodontal disease. In none of these areas do we have sufficient information on which to base national strategies for the control of periodontal disease.

European population data on periodontal disease are inadequate, both in relation to describing prevalences and as guidelines for the development of appropriate countermeasures. Further, the role of periodontal disease in tooth loss needs clarification.

Present day dental care in Europe for the adult populations is mainly based upon therapeutic/restorative measures aimed at the consequences of caries. However, in a number of countries, the dental professions have been active in the introduction of preventive measures for children and adolescents, a development which now bears fruit in the form of a notable decline in the prevalence of dental caries in these age groups.

The prospects for fewer carious teeth and more natural teeth retained in higher age groups call for a reconsideration of the orientation and procedures of dental care systems.

The failure of exclusively therapeutic measures in curbing disease activity is being recognized as is the need for shifting weight from cure to prevention – also in dental care for adults. It is, however, not at all clear what constitutes appropriate preventive dentistry for various groups of adult people. Effective secondary preventive programmes have been demonstrated in small groups of patients under close professional supervision, but so far there is no indication of how these principles may be implemented in large, less supervised groups.

Unless a 'one shot' miracle cure for periodontal disease (e.g. vaccination) is found, it appears that mass prevention and control must include self-assessment and self-care to a much higher degree than practiced hitherto. Methods by which this can be achieved are as badly needed as they are ill-defined.

Possibly, preventive dentistry might benefit from teaming up with other health sectors concerned with measures against the growing amount of chronic illnesses. Most of these are not lifethreatening, permitting people to provide themselves with some health care without professional help.

There is growing evidence (from general medical practice) that people with these types of diseases have already begun self-prescribed treatment prior to visiting their physician, and that the treatment is beneficial in the majority of the cases.

Appropriate health education, supplying people with knowledge and incentives to control common illnesses themselves and to chose the best time to see a physician/dentist could improve the effectiveness of self-care as a health resource.

Only rarely do present dental care delivery systems have oral health related goals, and descriptions of service elements specifically directed at periodontal health problems are almost nonexistent. Among the prerequisites for such descriptions are the development of concepts concerning acceptable levels of gingival and periodontal disease as well as the number of teeth needed to satisfy physiological and social functions.

Goals and strategies for oral health are fundamental to the description of dental care systems, including quality and quantity of manpower. Several European nations are presently experiencing severe disproportions between the output of dental manpower and the demand for services. The surplus of manpower may in part be a function of the dental delivery systems in operation, but it is also evident that diminished need for treatment plays a role, and that this aspect will be even more accentuated in the future. It is high time that the dental manpower systems are scrutinized in light of the changing pattern of dental diseases and simultaneously that dental delivery systems be evaluated and modified in order to serve future oral health care needs of the populations in the best possible way.

Hopefully, the present proceedings will contribute to a better understanding of the problems involved in dental care for the European populations and stimulate development in appropriate directions.

Asger Frandsen
1984

Reference

1. *Efficacy of Treatment Procedures in Periodontics.*
   (Shanley, D. ed.) Quintessence, Chicago, 1980.

Contents

Workpapers

Contents

Group work

Group Reports and Recommendations

Plenum Discussion and Recommendations

Index

Workpapers

1. Prevalence of Periodontal Disease

David E. Barmes

The Oral Health programme of the World Health Organization established a global data bank as part of its epidemiology sub-programme, which commenced in 1967. In that bank for dental caries we have been able to demonstrate similarities and contrasts in 130 countries, as well as the changes occurring over the last 15 years. For periodontal conditions, we have data for only about 40 countries, and almost no data on trends.

The present global periodontal disease picture is based on data collected by using the indices developed during 1955 to 1965. The indices most commonly used were the Periodontal Index (PI) and those outlined in the first edition of Oral Health Surveys, Basic Methods Manual;[3] percentage of the population affected with gingivitis, calculus and advanced periodontal disease (%G, %C, %PD). Global maps for adults at 35–44 years, based on %PD and PI, and for 15–19 year olds, based on %C, demonstrate a generally lower prevalence of the disease in North America, Northern Europe, Australia and New Zealand, and moderate to high levels in Latin America, Africa and Asia, though with a number of exceptions within these broad groupings.

In a special activity[2], a comparative set of data was collected, using the OHI-S and PI indices. As a useful reference, that set of data is reproduced in Tables 1.1 to 1.7.

During 1973–1977 it became clear that there were certain deficiencies in available periodontal disease indices when used as epidemiological tools, both with respect to examiner variability and in failing to provide information of practical use for the planning and development of preventive or curative services. All the data comparisons, whether local community, national or international, tended to indicate just one simple but important fact, namely that good oral hygiene reduced the prevalence of plaque, gingivitis and calculus. There was a need to know more than that single fact.

In 1977, the WHO Scientific Group Meeting on Epidemiology, Etiology and Prevention of Periodontal Diseases[1] proposed a new survey method based on separate recordings of pockets, calculus and bleeding for a restricted number of teeth. After extensive field-testing this method has been accepted and we are now rapidly gathering more reliable data using the Community Periodontal Index of Treatment Needs (CPITN). By use of this index, it is likely that the earlier general picture of higher prevalence in developing than in industrialized countries will be confirmed, as well as the indications that the difference represents a change in the latter as a result of better oral hygiene methods and programmes. However, it is also hoped that data generated by this method will go much further in quantifying differ-

Table 1.1   Mean scores for oral hygiene index and gingivitis (child sample 8−9-years-old).

Study area		OHI(S)	% Children free of gingivitis	Number of teeth with gingivitis
Baltimore	Metro	0.9	2	5.8
	Non-metro	0.7	3	4.5
Canterbury	Metro	0.9	0	6.4
	Non-metro	0.7	0	6.7
Dublin	Metro	1.6	2	7.5
	Non-metro	1.9	3	6.1
Hannover	Metro	1.5	2	8.5
	Non-metro	1.4	0	10.0
Leipzig	Metro	1.0	7	7.4
	Non-metro	1.0	0	10.3
Lodz	Metro	1.2	0	7.2
	Non-metro	1.2	1	8.4
Ontario	Metro	1.0	18	3.9
	Non-metro	0.9	18	3.4
Sydney	Metro	1.5	0	8.2
	Non-metro	1.4	0	9.2
Trondelag	Metro	1.3	0	8.9
	Non-metro	1.3	0	7.4
Yamanashi	Metro	1.8	2	5.2
	Non-metro	1.5	0	7.3

Table 1.2   Oral hygiene status (student sample 13−14-years-old).

Study area		Debris	Mean Scores Calculus	OHI(S)[1]
Alberta	Metro	0.7	0.1	0.7
	Non-metro	0.7	0.1	0.7
Baltimore	Metro	0.8	0.1	0.9
	Non-metro	0.7	0.0	0.8
Canterbury	Metro	0.7	0.0	0.7
	Non-metro	0.6	0.0	0.6
Dublin	Metro	1.3	0.4	1.7
	Non-metro	1.5	0.4	1.9
Hannover	Metro	1.2	0.0	1.2
	Non-metro	1.2	0.1	1.2
Leipzig	Metro	0.8	0.0	0.8
	Non-metro	0.8	0.0	0.8

Study area		Debris	Mean Scores Calculus	OHI(S)[1]
Lodz	Metro	0.9	0.2	1.1
	Non-metro	1.0	0.3	1.3
Ontario	Metro	0.7	0.1	0.9
	Non-metro	0.7	0.1	0.8
Quebec	Metro	1.0	0.2	1.1
	Non-metro	1.2	0.1	1.3
Sydney	Metro	1.1	0.0	1.1
	Non-metro	1.1	0.0	1.1
Trondelag	Metro	0.9	0.0	0.9
	Non-metro	1.0	0.0	1.0
Yamanashi	Metro	1.3	0.2	1.5
	Non-metro	1.3	0.2	1.5

[1] The debris and calculus scores may not add to OHI(S) because of rounding.

Table 1.3 Number of teeth with gingivitis and mean periodontal index (student sample 13–14-years-old).

Study area		Mean number teeth with gingivitis	Mean periodontal index	% with no gingivitis	% with periodontal index > 1.0
Alberta	Metro	14.1	0.65	1.4	36.9
	Non-metro	13.9	0.64	1.3	37.4
Baltimore	Metro	12.6	0.47	2.9	1.2
	Non-metro	12.4	0.45	2.0	2.0
Canterbury	Metro	13.4	0.53	0.0	1.3
	Non-metro	14.7	0.56	0.2	1.0
Dublin	Metro	14.2	0.55	0.6	1.8
	Non-metro	12.7	0.53	2.9	7.7
Hannover	Metro	17.6	0.75	0.0	21.6
	Non-metro	18.8	0.80	0.0	24.5
Leipzig	Metro	15.3	0.65	6.5	13.4
	Non-metro	19.5	0.92	0.4	34.9
Lodz	Metro	14.5	0.61	0.0	13.3
	Non-metro	18.6	0.89	0.0	34.6
Ontario	Metro	6.5	0.26	13.2	1.2
	Non-metro	6.6	0.26	17.0	1.1
Quebec	Metro	10.5	0.44	6.3	7.3
	Non-metro	10.7	0.46	4.3	8.2

Study area		Mean number teeth with gingivitis	Mean periodontal index	% with no gingivitis	% with periodontal index > 1.0
Sydney	Metro	16.7	0.75	0.2	22.0
	Non-metro	17.4	0.79	0.6	27.3
Trondelag	Metro	14.3	0.55	0.2	2.1
	Non-metro	13.6	0.53	0.4	2.2
Yamanashi	Metro	10.3	0.41	1.1	2.1
	Non-metro	17.1	0.71	0.3	15.1

Table 1.4 Periodontal treatment needs (student sample 13–14-years-old).

Study area			% of students requiring	
		Plaque removal	Major scaling	Recontouring/ replacing of restorations
Alberta	Metro	20	1	0
	Non-metro	26	1	0
Baltimore	Metro	15	1	0
	Non-metro	10	2	0
Canterbury	Metro	11	0	0
	Non-metro	17	0	0
Dublin	Metro	64	1	1
	Non-metro	54	2	11
Hannover	Metro	16	0	0
	Non-metro	18	1	0
Leipzig	Metro	79	0	0
	Non-metro	91	0	0
Lodz	Metro	22	7	3
	Non-metro	25	14	2
Ontario	Metro	56	3	0
	Non-metro	49	3	0
Quebec	Metro	44	1	0
	Non-metro	39	1	0
Sydney	Metro	31	0	0
	Non-metro	33	0	0
Trondelag	Metro	6	0	2
	Non-metro	11	0	3
Yamanashi	Metro	34	3	0
	Non-metro	43	2	2

Table 1.5 Oral hygiene status (adult sample 35−44-years-old).

Study area			Mean Scores	
		Debris	Calculus	OHI(S)[1]
Baltimore	Metro	0.6	0.8	1.4
	Non-metro	0.5	0.5	0.9
Canterbury	Metro	0.6	0.2	0.8
	Non-metro	0.6	0.2	0.8
Dublin	Metro	1.1	1.4	2.5
	Non-metro	1.2	1.4	2.5
Hannover	Metro	1.0	0.7	1.7
	Non-metro	1.0	0.7	1.7
Leipzig	Metro	0.6	0.3	0.9
	Non-metro	0.7	0.3	1.0
Lodz	Metro	0.8	1.1	1.9
	Non-metro	0.8	1.0	1.8
Ontario	Metro	0.8	0.9	1.7
	Non-metro	0.6	0.8	1.5
Sydney	Metro	0.8	0.2	1.0
	Non-metro	0.9	0.3	1.2
Trondelag	Metro	0.6	0.4	1.0
	Non-metro	0.6	0.6	1.2
Yamanashi	Metro	1.1	0.9	2.0
	Non-metro	1.1	1.0	2.1

[1] The debris and calculus scores may not add to OHI(S) because of rounding.

Table 1.6 Number of teeth with gingivitis and mean periodontal index (adult sample 35−44-years-old).

Study area		Mean number of teeth scored for PI	Mean number of teeth with gingivitis[1]	Mean PI	% with PI greater than 2
Baltimore	Metro	20.4	19.0	2.04	18.9
	Non-metro	21.4	18.2	1.61	9.4
Canterbury	Metro	22.5	16.8	0.99	2.8
	Non-metro	22.0	16.4	0.95	1.0
Dublin	Metro	19.8	12.8	1.02	8.4
	Non-metro	20.6	12.0	0.94	7.2
Hannover	Metro	24.2	22.3	1.73	29.5
	Non-metro	24.4	22.4	1.72	26.4

Study area		Mean number of teeth scored for PI	Mean number of teeth with gingivitis[1]	Mean PI	% with PI greater than 2
Leipzig	Metro	25.4	22.0	1.33	5.4
	Non-metro	24.6	21.7	1.43	9.0
Lodz	Metro	19.6	18.7	2.34	66.4
	Non-metro	15.5	15.0	2.41	75.6
Ontario	Metro	23.9	12.9	0.84	7.4
	Non-metro	22.1	12.5	0.81	5.0
Sydney	Metro	21.9	15.1	1.19	14.0
	Non-metro	19.2	13.5	1.26	15.9
Trondelag	Metro	22.6	14.4	0.96	6.9
	Non-metro	20.7	14.1	1.05	7.3
Yamanashi	Metro	26.2	24.0	1.60	18.3
	Non-metro	25.8	24.3	1.86	34.5

[1] Mean number of teeth with gingivitis includes teeth with scores 1, 2, 3, 6 and 8.

Table 1.7 Periodontal treatment needs (adult sample 35–44-years-old).

Study area		% of adults by category		
		Plaque removal	Major scaling	Recontouring/ replacing restorations
Baltimore	Metro	28	41	9
	Non-metro	37	20	10
Canterbury	Metro	28	7	0
	Non-metro	20	9	0
Dublin	Metro	47	43	15
	Non-metro	48	34	31
Hannover	Metro	54	27	0
	Non-metro	60	26	0
Leipzig	Metro	82	7	2
	Non-metro	90	8	0
Lodz	Metro	12	81	3
	Non-metro	17	71	0
Ontario	Metro	79	40	4
	Non-metro	67	28	3

Study area		Plaque removal	Major scaling	Recontouring/ replacing restorations
			% of adults by category	
Sydney	Metro	56	13	2
	Non-metro	45	13	0
Trondelag	Metro	49	19	18
	Non-metro	45	26	27
Yamanashi	Metro	55	32	19
	Non-metro	50	44	23

Table 1.8 CPITN sextant score ranges at 15 years of age.

Countries	B[1]	C[2]	P1[3]
France	1.9	1.1	
Norway	2.0	0.8	
Sweden	2.5	1.5	
Syria	2.7	1.6	
Emro Refugees	3.9	3.4	
Italy	4.2	2.8	
Tonga	4.9	3.7	0.7
Philippines	5.0	2.7	
South Korea	5.2	3.6	0.2
Western Samoa	5.3	4.0	0.1
China	3.8	3.5	0.3
Morocco	3.0	1.9	0.0

[1] B = bleeding
[2] C = calculus
[3] P1 = periodontal pockets of 4 or 5 mm (prepared at WHO 1982)

Table 1.9 Service requirements ranges at 15 years of age.

Countries	TN1[1] % of persons	TN2[2] % of persons	SEXT[3]
France	68	57	(0.1)
Norway	80	45	
Syria	81	67	(1.6)
Emro Refugees	95	86	(3.4)
Italy	98	93	(2.8)
Bangladesh	96	82	(3.4)
Philippines	97	73	
Tonga	97	81	
South Korea	98	92	
Western Samoa	100	95	
Morocco	85	72	(3.0)

[1] TN1 = oral hygiene instruction
[2] TN2 = scaling
[3] SEXT = sextant (prepared at WHO 1982)

ences between populations for the various factors measured, in terms of treatment need and, thus, in giving much greater precision to planning preventive and other services.

Tables 1.8 to 1.11 present the first sets of data using CPITN. Although country names have been used in these tables, the data presented in most cases relates to special samples which are not necessarily representative of whole populations.

Table 1.10 CPITN sextant score ranges at 35 years of age.

Countries	B[1]	C[2]	P1[3]	P2[4]
France	2.3	1.4	0.3	0.0
South Korea (ama)	2.6	2.3	0.0	0.0
South Korea	5.4	4.7	0.9	0.3
Philippines	5.6	4.4	0.4	0.0
Tonga	5.7	5.5	4.4	1.4
Western Samoa	5.9	5.7	2.7	0.7
Bangladesh	6.0	5.7	5.2	1.2

[1] B = bleeding
[2] C = calculus
[3] P1 = periodontal pockets of 4 or 5 mm
[4] P2 = periodontal pockets of 6 or more mm (prepared at WHO, 1982)

It can be seen, by comparing data from developed and developing countries, that developing countries have much higher levels of bleeding and calculus, but not necessarily higher levels of pocketing at an early age. This first set of data also reveals some fundamental contrasts within the developing countries represented in terms of prevalence of pocketing, the differences being quite marked, even though prevalence of bleeding and calculus in adults and at the younger age group are similar.

These indications are preliminary and must be studied further. However, the signs are good that we will soon have a much better data base by which to measure differences and trends, and a reliable tool to use for monitoring and evaluation of preventive programmes.

Our task is now to develop strategies for implementation of prevention and control programmes for periodontal diseases. While it is possible to provide information to whole populations on oral hygiene, specific instruction to all groups is well nigh impossible in even the richest of countries. Similarly, it is not likely that scaling can be provided for all who have calculus and, thus, there is a need to investigate different criteria for defining the various treatment-need categories, and priority groups within these categories, as a parallel activity to developing really effective oral hygiene instruction methods. For example, should oral hygiene instruction (TN1) be given only to individuals who have more than two bleeding sextants or only to those with more than four? Similar decisions are needed regarding the provision of scaling (TN2) – Whom to scale? In how many sessions or stages? When and how much? – need to be made before economically feasible and acceptable programmes can be developed.

Table 1.11 Service requirements ranges at 35 years of age.

Countries	TN1[1] % of persons	TN2[2] % of persons	SEXT[4]	TN3[3] % of persons	SEXT[4]
South Korea (ama)	86	80	(2.3)	0	(0.0)
Philippines	100	94	(4.4)	0	(0.0)
Bangladesh	100	100	(5.7)	0.5	(1.2)
France	76	66	(1.4)	3	(0.0)
South Korea	100	100	(4.7)	28	(0.3)
Western Samoa	100	100	(5.7)	36	(0.7)
Tonga	100	100	(5.5)	47	(1.4)

[1] TN1 = oral hygiene instruction
[2] TN2 = scaling
[3] TN3 = complex periodontal care
[4] SEXT = sextant (prepared at WHO 1982)

As the data bank using CPITN expands, we hope to be able to provide information on the relevance of different strategies being applied.

Though not strictly part of the subject, an annex to this paper has been included to provide an outline for an evaluation of community periodontal control and prevention programmes that were proposed as part of the second stage of the FDI/WHO Joint Working Group on Integrated Planning of Oral Health Services, with special attention to periodontal diseases. Evaluation of this sort of programme will be fundamental to our future appreciation of prevalence data in relation to periodontal disease.

References

1. Epidemiology, etiology and prevention of periodontal diseases. Techn. Rep. Ser. 1978. 621, Geneva.

2. International Collaborative Study of Dental Manpower Systems in Relation to Oral Health Status. Final Report. FDI/WHO. 1984. (In press).

3. Oral Health Surveys. Basic Methods, 2nd ed. WHO, Geneva. 1977.

4. Development of the World Health Organization (WHO) Community Periodontal Index of Treatment Needs (CPITN) Int. dent. J. 1982. 32 (3): 281–291.

Annex: Evaluation of Community Periodontal Control and Preventive Programmes

Following the WHO Scientific Group Meeting on *Epidemiology, Etiology and Prevention of Periodontal Diseases,* held in November/December 1977, a successful methodology testing operation has been carried out by a Joint Working Group of the FDI/WHO. It is now proposed that this collaboration should continue using the methodology thus developed, and the philosophy for management of periodontal disease accepted at the 1977 meeting, to implement and evaluate community periodontal control and preventive programmes.

General Description

Programmes should be designed as de-monstration or pilot projects which, if successful, will then become a permanent part of the country's preventive health services and will serve as a model for expansion of the programme to other parts of the population. Proposed projects must be compatible with existing services and use personnel, materials and treatment available in the country. Except for initial training, monitoring and programme evaluation phases, projects will not depend on imported personnel.

The implementation of these projects will depend on the following:

1. Satisfactory definition of methodology which is applicable, or adaptable to all the populations being included in the project for:

29

(a) assessment of oral health status and periodontal treatment needs. (CPITN) (Use of radiographs may be possible at some project sites.)

(b) describing and characterizing the population in terms of socioeconomic levels, education levels, exposure to mass media and any existing health education programmes (percentage of people who have radio, TV, read newspapers, attend health clinics, etc.), and the present level of demand for oral care for both caries and periodontal diseases (to be obtained from a review of public health services and private practice records indicating the existing level and extent of care).

2. Design and preparation of appropriate materials and methods for:

(a) sensitizing and re-orientating existing personnel, and training new personnel involved in the project (teaching materials for dentists, auxiliaries and primary health workers, for reorientation, basic training and for in-service training);

(b) convincing people to care for and seek care for their periodontal tissues (materials for TV, radio, newspapers, posters, etc., for distribution in schools, health centres, cinemas, markets, work places, etc.). These materials will probably be specific for each country but will provide materials for use in countries of similar cultural backgrounds.

Possible participating countries

Preference will be given to developing countries: industrialized countries will be included in the project if feasible.

A stable community (rural or peri-urban) is required. The whole of the adult population of the community will be included in the programme. It will therefore be necessary to choose villages and/or towns of sizes appropriate to the programme personnel available and projected, and sufficiently isolated from each other to maintain different régimes.

The project should identify the following:

1. Preventive approaches which are effective in different populations.
2. Public relations or oral health education programmes which are successful.
3. Whether there is a critical age or severity after which it is not feasible to control periodontal diseases as part of a public health programme.
4. Effective training materials for oral disease prevention for all levels of personnel.
5. Whether destructive periodontal disease can be prevented by commencing prevention at 15–19 years of age.
6. Average treatment times for procedures performed by various personnel in different environments.

It is envisaged that the project would be centrally coordinated by a dentist with postgraduate training and teaching experience. A steering committee of experienced public health administrators/periodontists will assist FDI/WHO in the overall administration and monitoring of the project and serve as consultants as needed. In each country there will be an administrator (dentist), probably from the Department of Health, who will be responsible for the project organization and staff. Care will be provided by local health personnel and, depending on the actual study design, may include dentists (either in private practice or in government employment), auxiliaries and nondental health workers.

The Programme Coordinator, together with a member of the steering committee, would be responsible for negotiating the establishment of the project with the Ministry of Health in each country. The projects will use the CPITN methodology and incorporate in varying patterns and combinations the following parameters:

1. *Oral Hygiene Education*
   (a) A community-based programme.
   (b) Individual or small group instruction.
2. *Personnel*
   (a) Dentists and nondental personnel only.
   (b) Dentists and dental auxiliaries and oral health education personnel.
   (c) Specialists, dentists, dental auxiliaries and oral health education personnel.
3. *Care Patterns*
   (a) No initial care, no formal recall.
   (b) Initial care and no formal recall.
   (c) Initial care and formal fixed term recall.
   (d) Initial care and selective recall.

Only the following three types of services are envisaged in any of the designs combining the above parameters:

1. Individual oral health education (OHE).
2. Scaling.
3. Complex therapy (includes deep scaling and surgery, also extractions).

Study Designs

Designs A–G below present combinations of services and personnel most likely to occur in participating countries. They are to be used in identifying possible study sites; it is intended that only a few of these designs will be selected for the project. It is also possible that other combinations could replace those suggested. The definitive plan would be available only after site visits. The proposed designs are:

A. 1. No community oral hygiene education programme (COHEP). OHE, scaling and complex therapy provided on demand by dentists.

2. No COHEP. OHE and scaling provided by auxiliaries and complex therapy provided by dentists on demand.
3. COHEP. OHE, scaling and complex therapy provided on demand by dentists.
4. COHEP. OHE and scaling provided by auxiliaries and complex therapy provided by dentists on demand.

B. Community oral hygiene education programmes are provided to all groups, patients can be referred for more complicated therapy, initial care (oral hygiene instruction and removal of deposits) is provided to all at the start of the project and thereafter on demand.

1. OHE and scaling provided by nondental personnel.
2. OHE and scaling provided by dental auxiliaries.
3. OHE, scaling and complex therapy provided by dentists.

C. Community oral hygiene education programmes are provided to all groups, patients can be referred for more complicated therapy, initial care is provided to all at the start of the project and thereafter on demand.

1. OHE and scaling provided by nondental personnel
2. OHE, scaling and complex therapy provided by dentists

D. Community oral hygiene education programmes are provided to all groups, patients can be referred for more complicated treatment, initial care is provided to all at the start of the project and thereafter at fixed intervals.

1. OHE and scaling provided by nondental personnel
2. OHE and scaling provided by dental auxiliaries

31

3. OHE, scaling and complex therapy provided by dentists.

E. Replicate of D 1 and 3 in countries where dental auxiliaries do not exist.

F. Community oral hygiene education programmes are provided to all groups and patients can be referred for more complex therapy. Nondental personnel provide OHE, and scaling is provided by auxiliaries.

1. Initial care and fixed term recall.
2. Initial care and selective recall.

G. Community oral hygiene education programmes are provided to all groups and patients can be referred for more complicated therapy. Nondental personnel provide OHE and scaling is provided by dentists.

1. Initial care and fixed term recall.
2. Initial care and selective recall.

NB. Any of these designs may, or may not, include specialists for the referral system.

Implementation

In any one country the sequence of activities will be initial and periodic.

Initial

1. Identification of interest at national (health ministry) level.
2. Identification of responsible administrators and appropriate population groups.
3. Negotiations with commercial companies active in the country regarding the

design and production of oral hygiene education materials.
4. Inventory of oral health personnel available and expected, facilities of possible use for the project (health centres, work sites, etc) and media in use in the population.
5. Decisions, in agreement with local administrators, as to the range and type of preventive/maintenance care, and the study groups to be used.
6. Description and characterization of the population in terms of socio-economic demographic measures, exposure to various media and use of health care facilities.
7. Development of training/sensitizing or reorientating courses needed for oral health and other personnel.
8. Design, field/pilot testing and production of oral hygiene education materials in collaboration with the media.
9. Implementation of training/re-orientating courses for all personnel who will be involved in the programme, including teaching personnel.
10. Baseline examination of subjects.
11. Commencement of actual programme.

Periodic

1. In-service courses for local staff (annually).
2. Design and production of new oral hygiene education material (as needed).
3. Monitoring of project activities (annually).
4. Evaluation of oral health status at 1, 3 and 5 years.

NB. It should be noted that the evaluation after 1 year is more an assessment of feasibility and acceptance of the system than an evaluation of change in oral health status.

2. Assessment of Periodontal Treatment Needs: Adaptation of the WHO Community Periodontal Index of Treatment Needs (CPITN) to European Countries

Jukka Ainamo

Introduction

An important aim of epidemiological research is to describe the prevalence of a given disease and to determine its aetiology. For periodontal diseases, these questions have been given substantial attention during the past 30 years. In the 1950s the first indices for measurement of periodontal disease were developed.[41, 45] The early descriptive studies linked periodontal disease with a number of demographic and social factors. Periodontal disease of greater severity was recorded in men than in women, in black than in white people, in rural than in urban populations. Also, periodontal disease is associated with level of education, age and oral hygiene.

After the introduction of reliable epidemiological indices for the measurement of oral hygiene levels,[20, 21, 40, 41, 50] the demographic and social factors were found to be a reflection of the population's oral hygiene behaviour.[19, 30, 47, 51, 52] During the 1960s it was thus possible to take the final step in the clarification of the aetiology of periodontal disease. In controlled clinical studies it was demonstrated that proper oral hygiene measures, combined with subgingival scaling, reduce gingivitis,[33] that undisturbed colonization of plaque on the tooth surfaces resulted in gingivitis and that gingivitis may or may not develop into progressive periodontitis, i.e. irreversible loss of tooth attachment.[29]

During the 1970s the main emphasis was on attempts to assess the value of various treatment modalities for dealing with the problem of periodontitis.[43, 44] At the same time, concern was expressed about the slow implementation of the acquired knowledge for the benefit of the general public.[6]

The transition period from descriptive surveys to controlled clinical trials included constant refinement of the criteria used for measurement of disease. Eventually the diagnostic tools by far surpassed applicability in daily dental practice, both with regard to the ability of the general practitioner and to the time required for recording. It became increasingly evident that a simple and rapid scoring system was badly needed for the assessment of periodontal treatment needs in the daily work of the dental practitioner.

Assessment of Periodontal Treatment Needs

A study of the available literature reveals an abundance of information about the severity of periodontal disease in various populations. The results have been obtained through determination of the mean of the scores of all teeth[45] or of selected index teeth[41] of the individual, and then by calculating the mean of all individual means recorded in the study population. Such data have been very useful for comparison of periodontal disease levels in different parts of the world. Mean severity scores, however, give no information about the actual proportion of individuals affected within the population.

The prevalence of periodontal disease specifically refers to the proportion of subjects affected by periodontal disease or various degrees of it. Although such data could be produced using almost any index system, they have rarely been published. In the exceptionally thorough review on *The Epidemiology of Gingival and Periodontal Disease*[11] there is only one reference on prevalence of periodontal disease in adults.[26] This study gives the exact and valuable information that in the USA about 25% of adults 18 to 79 years of age had destructive periodontal disease.[26] This is the type of information a public health administrator would need for planning purposes.

The dental practitioner's main interest is to determine, with simple criteria and in the shortest possible time, the periodontal treatment needs of the patient seated in the chair. For this purpose most of the early epidemiological indices are too complicated and time-consuming. *Russell's Periodontal Index*[45] requires scoring of all teeth while *Ramfjord's Periodontal Disease Index*[41] as well as *O'Leary's Gingivo-Periodontal Index*[37] do not measure pocket depth but loss of attachment which is not necessarily an indication of treatment needs. The amount of permanent loss of tooth attachment would in the majority of cases be the same after as before treatment. Several of the indices used, for example, the *GPI*,[37] the *Oral Hygiene Index*,[20] the *Gingival and Plaque Indices*,[31] and the *Gingival Sulcus Bleeding Index*[35] involve determination of several degrees of severity of various disease indicators. It is not likely that the practising dentist would ever adopt such scoring procedures.

Comparison between different methods

A number of analyses have been published in which a close correlation has been demonstrated between the many different methods for determining mean severity of periodontal disease.[16, 18, 24, 28, 34, 46, 48, 49] At the same time, however, it has been clearly realized that severity scores do not give adequate information about the prevalence and treatment needs of the disease.[4, 23, 36, 42] Calculation of conversion factors has from time-to-time been suggested to enable the use of mean severity scores for assessment of treatment needs.[18, 42] Such an approach might be of value in the assessment of, for example, national manpower needs, but would not contribute to the important identification of those individuals who are affected the worst.

Since difficulties have also been experienced in efforts to calibrate investigators to use the classical epidemiological indices,[15] it seems justified to conclude that traditional assessments of periodontal disease, although valuable for comparing one population with another, represent rather crude methods from the viewpoint of determining treatment needs.

Most of the methods designed for assessment of periodontal treatment needs have been constructed by specialist periodontists who seem to have had difficulties in differentiating between a rapid survey methodology and the painstakingly detailed examination required for performing the actual treatment procedures. In most cases the result has been something in between these two goals. Without exception, the gain in accuracy of recording has meant a loss in terms of time needed for recording. The determination and recording of plaque and calculus alone requires 2 + 2 minutes,[20] whereas buccally performed measurement of pocket depth mesially and distally of each tooth takes about 5 minutes.[39] With more complicated recording systems the time required for scoring treatment needs may total 25 minutes.[10, 12]

Simplified assessments of treatment needs

The requirements of periodontal indices for prevalence studies have been defined by Davies[14] as follows:

1. It should be simple to use and should permit the study of a large number of persons in a minimum time and at minimum cost.
2. The criteria which define the components of an index should be clear, readily understandable and promote diagnostic reproducibility both within and between examiners.
3. It should be amenable to statistical analysis.
4. If it is used to describe severity, the index should be equally sensitive throughout the scale and should indicate in a meaningful way the clinical stages in the disease process.

It is of interest to notice that at least a few studies that more or less conform to these requirements have been published by nonperiodontists whose main interest has been to describe the situation rather than make preparations for carrying out the treatment[8, 13]
Simplification of the periodontal examination was suggested by *Ramfjord*[41] and by *Greene* and *Vermillion*[21] who chose to examine and record the findings from only one representative tooth in each of the four posterior and two anterior segments of the dentition. *O'Leary* further developed this idea by suggesting examination of all teeth, but recording of only the worst condition in each segment.[37, 38] In this index, however, several degrees of severity still were to be determined separately for gin-

givitis, loss of tooth attachment, and soft and hard deposits.[37]
The next important step towards simplification of the recording of periodontal treatment needs was taken when the *Periodontal Treatment Need System* (PTNS) was published in the early 1970s.[25] The PTNS represented at that time a most untraditional approach which may be one reason why it never gained very wide usage. Instead of scoring various disease indicators, the PTNS was designed to directly measure the need for periodontal surgery, scaling and oral hygiene instructions. A code is given to each one of the four quadrants of the dentition. The three types of treatment needs can further be added up by using the time needed per quadrant for the type of treatment indicated. After actual treatment of the patients examined, the average times arrived at for each patient was 60 minutes for oral hygiene education, 30 minutes per quadrant for scaling and 60 minutes per quadrant for periodontal surgery.[25] In a subsequent study of 35-year-old citizens in Oslo, only about 2% were found not to need treatment, about 8% were found to need only motivation and instruction in oral hygiene measures whereas over 50% were in need of scaling and about 40% needed combined surgery and scaling.[22] Both the percentage needing professional care and the time needed for treatment were somewhat lower when a different approach was utilized by *Ekanayaka* and *Sheiham*.[17, 18]
The third step towards simplified recording of periodontal disorders was the proposal by *Ainamo* and *Bay*[6] to score only presence or absence of visible plaque and of a gingival bleeding tendency. Bleeding may be provoked in primary school children by applying pressure to the gingival margin or, in adolescents and adults, by gentle probing of the pockets. The principle of simple dichotomous recording was subsequently expanded to include also other periodontal disease indicators.[2] Dichotomous criteria, if carefully chosen,

35

were suggested to improve the reproducibility of recordings[14] and also to simplify subsequent data processing.[6]

A combination of the sextant approach by O'Leary et al.,[38] the PTNS[25] and the principle of using dichotomous criteria for periodontal disease indicators[6] resulted in the development of the *Community Periodontal Index of Treatment Needs*[5] which was explicitly designed for rapid assessment of both prevalence and treatment needs of periodontal disorders.

The Community Periodontal Index of Treatment Needs (CPITN)

The Community Periodontal Index (CPI) was developed in collaboration between the Federation Dentaire Internationale (FDI) and the Oral Health Unit of the World Health Organization (WHO). A description of the methodology has been published by *Ainamo et al.*[5] Subsequent slight adjustments to that description are indicated here with an asterisk.

Sextants

The periodontal treatment needs are recorded for sextants, i.e. 6ths of the dentition. Third molars are not included, except where they are functioning in the place of second molars. The sextants contain the following teeth:

17−14	13−23	24−27
47−44	43−33	34−37

The treatment need in a sextant is recorded only when 2 or more teeth are present and not indicated for extraction. The indication for extraction because of periodontal involvement is that the tooth has vertical mobility and causes discomfort to the patient. If only one functioning tooth remains in a sextant, it is included in the adjoining sextant. For example, if only 2 teeth remained in the maxilla, the jaw would be recorded as one sextant only. Missing sextants are indicated with a cross in the appropriate box*.

Use of index teeth

epidemiological surveys

In epidemiological surveys assessing the periodontal treatment needs of a population, the recordings per sextant are based on findings from specified index teeth. The index teeth to be examined are:

17,16	11	26,27
47,46	31	36,37

Although 10 index teeth are examined, only 6 recordings, one relating to each sextant, are made. When both or one of the designated molar teeth are present, the worst finding from these tooth surfaces is recorded for the sextant. If no index teeth are present in a sextant qualifying for examination, all the remaining teeth in that sextant are examined.

In large surveys, the findings in every 10th or 20th subject should be recorded both by examination of the designated index teeth and by the worst finding per sextant *(see below)* so that the results obained by partial examination can be subjected to analysis of reliability. An underestimate of up to 20% can be expected in the identification of adults with advanced periodontal disease (see Code 4, p. 39).

Correspondingly, an overestimate of deep pockets will occur in children and adolescents unless false recordings of pathological pocket depth, in particular at erupting teeth are avoided.

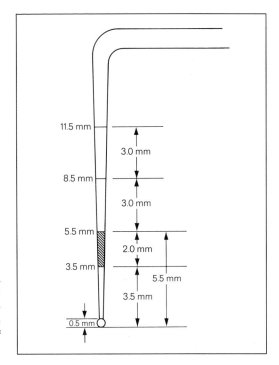

Fig. 2.1 The WHO periodontal probe has a 'ball-tip' end for easier detection of subgingival calculus and to avoid false reading by over-measurement. The colour shaded area from 3.5 to 5.5 mm greatly facilitates rapid reading of pocket depth.[53]

Recording of worst finding per sextant

Individual patient care

In oral health screening examinations for the determination of treatment needs of *individual patients,* where partial recording using index teeth would prove insufficient, the recording for each sextant is based on the worst finding from all teeth in that sextant. This screening method is suitable for use in comprehensive dental care systems for adult populations with a history of high caries prevalence and extensive restorative treatment. Hence, this approach would thus specifically apply to most European countries.

For age groups under 20 years, full sextant recordings have little advantage over partial recordings. At ages 7–19 years the recommendation is to base the recordings on clinical findings from the upper right and lower left incisor in the anterior sextants and on findings from the first molars in the posterior sextants*:

16	11	26
46	31	36

The WHO periodontal examination probe

For simple recording of the periodontal treatment needs, the use of the WHO probe is recommended.[53] The instrument was designed for two purposes: namely, measurement of pocket depth and detection of subgingival calculus. The pocket depth is measured through colour coding of the WHO probe, with a black mark starting at 3.5 mm and ending at 5.5 mm (Fig.

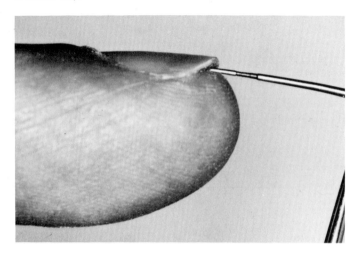

Fig. 2.2 The recommended force, corresponding to 20–25 g, should cause no pain to the examinee during probing procedure. A practical test for establishing this force is to probe underneath the finger nail where the sensitivity approximates that of the bottom of a periodontal pocket.[5]

2.1). The probe has a 'ball tip' of 0.5 mm that allows easy detection of subgingival calculus. The ball tip also facilitates the identification of the base of the pocket, thus decreasing the tendency for false reading by over-measurement.

It is realized that the use of any pocket probe does not provide the clinician with accurate measurements of pockets in millimetres which, even if feasible, are of doubtful value. Instead, the probe measures what is 'normal' and 'abnormal' with indications of treatment requirements being derived from 'abnormal' scores. A force of no more than 20–25 g is considered sufficient to reveal pathology without causing pain to the subject.

The probing procedure

A tooth is probed to determine pocket depth and to detect calculus and bleeding response. The probing force can be divided into a working component to determine pocket depth, and a sensing component to detect subgingival calculus. A practical test for establishing the working force of no more than 25 g is to gently insert the probe point under the finger nail (Fig. 2.2) without causing pain or discomfort. When inserting the probe into a periodontal pocket, the ballpoint should follow the anatomic configuration of the root surface. For sensing subgingival calculus, the lightest possible force which allows movement of the probe ballpoint along the tooth surface is used.

Pain to the patient during probing is in most cases indicative of the use of a too heavy probing force.

There is no rule specifying the number of separate probings to be made. This will depend on the condition of the tissues surrounding the teeth. However, when only the index tooth or teeth are being examined or when the recording is based on the worst finding in all teeth of the sextant, it would be rare to exceed four probings per sextant. Whenever available, radiographs will greatly enhance identification of advanced periodontal lesions.

Recording of findings

In assessing treatment needs, the presence of the following indicators is deter-

Fig. 2.3 The use of the WHO periodontal probe for determination of treatment needs. When the shaded coded area of the probe disappears into the pathologic pocket, the pocket depth is 6 mm or more and Code 4 is recorded, indicating the need for complex treatment. If the shaded coded area remains partially visible, pocket depth is either 4 or 5 mm and Code 3 is given. If there are no pocket depths exceeding 3 mm but calculus is present, the sextant is given Code 2. Codes 3 and 2 indicate a need for scaling. In the absence of pockets and calculus, the sextant is given Code 1 if bleeding occurs and Code 0 if bleeding does not occur after probing. Code 1 indicates the need for improved oral hygiene. Code 0 indicates no need for treatment.[5]

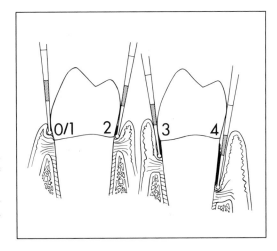

mined for each sextant in the sequence given below:

	Code
Pathologic pockets, 6 mm or deeper	4
Pathologic pockets, 4–5 mm deep	3
Supra- or subgingival calculus, defective margins of fillings or crowns	2
Gingival bleeding after gentle probing	1
Periodontal health	0

Whenever a 6 mm or deeper pocket is found at any designated tooth or teeth in the sextant being examined, a code of 4 is given to the sextant. Recording of Code 4 makes further examination of that sextant unnecessary. If the deepest pocket found at the designated tooth or teeth in a sextant is 4–5 mm, Code 3 is recorded. Again there is no further examination. If no pockets deeper than 3 mm are observed, the presence of supra- or subgingival calculus and/or overhangs of fillings or crowns is indicated by the recording of Code 2 for the sextant. If neither deep or moderate pocketing nor calculus is observed, but bleeding occurs after probing,

Code 1 is given to the sextant examined. The gingivae of the designated tooth or teeth should be inspected for the presence or absence of bleeding before the examinee is allowed to swallow or close his mouth. At times bleeding may be delayed for 10–30 seconds after probing. If the sextant is found healthy, Code 0 (zero) is given to the examined sextant. These codes are indicated diagrammatically in Fig. 2.3.

Classification of treatment needs

Subjects are classified into the different treatment need categories according to the highest score recorded during the examination. In epidemiological surveys this classification will be made automatically by the computer programme, according to the following rules.

Obviously, a recording of Code 0 (zero) for all six sextants indicates that there is no need for treatment. If codes of 1 are the only ones identified, the need for improvement in the personal oral hygiene of that individual is indicated. A maximum code of 2 indicates the need for professional debridement of the teeth. As moderate pocketing (4–5 mm, Code 3) can likewise be managed with a combination of professional and personal cleaning of the teeth, the treatment need is the same for Codes 2 and 3. Clearly, the patient also requires oral hygiene instruction.

A sextant scoring Code 4 (6 mm or deeper pockets) may or may not be successfully treated by means of deep scaling and efficient personal oral hygiene measures. Code 4 is therefore assigned to 'complex treatment' which may involve deep scaling and root planing under local anaesthesia, or require surgical exposure of the infected root surface in order to gain the access needed to clean it.

A subject or a sextant would thus be classified according to periodontal treatment need into one of the following treatment categories:

0   = No treatment (Code 0)
I   = Improvement in personal oral hygiene (Code 1)
II = I + scaling, removal of overhangs (Codes 2 and 3)
III = I + II + complex treatment (Code 4)

Examples of CPITN recordings: Treatment planning

The CPITN is designed for rapid and practical assessment of various periodontal treatment needs in population surveys and for initial screening of patients attending for regular dental care. For patients requiring oral hygiene instruction and scaling only, the CPITN recordings are sufficient for treatment planning. However, a finding of the need for complex treatment necessitates a more precise identification of the teeth and tooth surfaces affected before starting the actual therapy required by the individual patient.

It must be emphasized that the CPITN does not provide an assessment of past periodontal disease experience. It does not record the position of the gingival margin, that is, the degree of recession, and hence, except where pocketing is present, the level of the alveolar bone. These factors are relevant to the assessment of the overall periodontal condition (status) but they do not generally affect treatment need because they are not usually reversible (Fig. 2.4).

The time needed for the CPITN in recording the codes for the six segments should not exceed 1–2 minutes. The information obtained is illustrated by the following examples:

Case 1.

4	2	3
2	2	X

There is at least one deep pocket in the right posterior and one or more moderately deep pockets in the left posterior sextant of the maxilla. Three sextants have no pocket depths over 3 mm, but do require scaling. Apparently, the patient also needs oral hygiene instruction. One sextant is missing.

Case 2.

X	X	X
1	2	1

The maxilla is edentulous. The lower anterior sextant requires scaling. In addition, the patient requires instructions for improved personal oral hygiene.

Case 3.

3	0	4
4	1	4

There are deep or moderately deep pockets in all posterior sextants; there is a need for improved personal hygiene also in the lower anterior sextant and no treat-

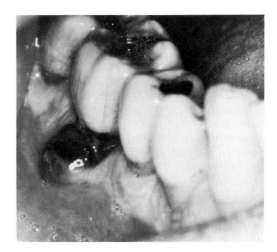

Fig. 2.4a   Prior to treatment there is a 7 mm deep pocket and abscess formation buccally on tooth 46. Code 4 is given to the sextant.

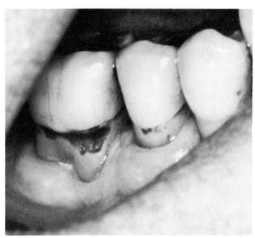

Fig. 2.4b   After deep scaling and a few weeks of proper oral hygiene, pocket depth is below 3 mm. There is no bleeding after probing. Code 0 is given to the sextant in spite of apparent loss of tooth attachment.

ment need in the upper anterior one. If this proved to be a young patient, the possibility of juvenile periodontitis should be considered.

Recall examinations after treatment

In countries where advanced periodontal treatment has become a regular part of oral health care, an increasing number of patients have had their deep inflamed periodontal pockets transformed into non-inflamed long epithelial attachments. For this reason, it has been argued that pocket depths, as assessed by probing, are not relevant to the determination of periodontal health or disease. The provision of optimal periodontal care being one of the main goals of dentistry, this statement deserves to be clarified.

The use of a standard force for probing is the most essential and critical part in the use of the CPITN or any other modern system for evaluation of periodontal health. The recommended 25 g is a very light force which will be resisted by a healthy epithelial attachment. It is important that the use of this force be thoroughly practised before starting the examination procedure. Various types of pressure-sensitive probes are already available for calibration purposes. A letter balance may also prove useful.

The use of the WHO probe with a 25 g force is in most cases sufficient for the detection of a re-infected long epithelial attachment and to elicit bleeding from the area of inflammation. Use of the standardized probing force thus maximizes the likelihood that only inflamed pockets are recorded. The sign of inflammation is bleeding after such probing.

Recall examinations and proper maintenance care have recently been demonstrated to be the major determinants of success or failure after treatment of advanced periodontal disease.[7]

Future Strategies

Compared to earlier systems for assessment of periodontal treatment needs, the CPI seems to offer many advantages. Even if a Code 4 patient needs additional examination for the actual treatment, this *need* is detected in 1–2 minutes and a new appointment time can be given for further charting of the precise number and location of deep pockets. If the patient is to be referred to another dentist for treatment, the CPI scorings are sufficient for that purpose. The short time required for recording the six CPI code numbers makes the system especially suitable for use at the diagnostic departments of dental schools and public dental health services. The advantage over the PTNS[25] is that some supragingival calculus on the lower anteriors will be recorded as one

sextant needing scaling according to the CPI whereas all teeth, i.e. both mandibular quadrants would have been assigned to scaling according to the PTNS. This difference is of particular value in the recording of treatment needs in children and adolescents.

Identification of high risk groups is also facilitated by the sextant approach. For the prevention of subsequent periodontal breakdown it would seem justified to give special attention to those school children who demonstrate a bleeding tendency in 5–6 sextants, whereas for a child with bleeding in only 0–2 sextants less rigid plaque control might well be sufficient. It has been suggested that children, when starting primary school, should be made aware of their bleeding gums and advised how to stop this bleeding.[3]

However, the CPI will not only be of benefit to children and public health services. It seems that private dental practitioners are the ones who most anxiously have been waiting for a simple and reliable method of screening their adult patients for periodontal disease. In some countries miniature CPI charts are already available on glued paper for insertion into the patient record whenever a baseline or a maintenance care examination is made. For this purpose the use of whole mouth examination is essential as the risk of not identifying the individual patient is greatest with regard to Code 4, i.e. the most severe state of periodontal disease.[4]

The relevance of all these considerations to the development of future strategies for European periodontal care is that current information about periodontal treatment needs is practically non-existent. Every effort should be made to gather more data. In school dental services and subsidized dental care systems for adults it would help to put the salaried dentists under the obligation to provide administrators with annual recordings. This approach would serve the purpose of monitoring the changes occurring in prevalence and treatment needs of periodontal disease.[1] Description of the individual's periodontal disease status with only 6 digits per person makes data processing a relatively easy task.

In the not too distant future, computerized charting of patient records will also become a common procedure in the office of the general dental practitioner. By then, it should be possible for administrators and health services planners to draw information from all parts of the country and to utilize this information for quantitative and qualitative assessment of needs for further dental health personnel.

An educated guess would be that about one-third of the adult population of Europe has advanced periodontal disease. Whether this guess is right or wrong is a question which deserves high priority in the health research of the next few years. Periodontal disease is a most unpleasant condition to the individual patient. The next step would thus be to provide proper periodontal treatment and adequate maintenance care to the parents and grandparents of those children and adolescents whose improved dental health many European countries are currently announcing with great pride.

References

1. *Ainamo J.*
   The monitoring process and its importance. Int. Dent. J., 1983, 33: 79–89.

2. *Ainamo J.* and *Ainamo A.*
   Development of oral health during dental studies in India and Finland. Int. Dent. J., 1978, 28: 427–433.

3. *Ainamo J.* and *Ainamo A.*
   Prevention of periodontal disease in the mixed dentition. Int. Dent. J., 1981, 31: 125–132.

4. *Ainamo J.* and *Ainamo A.*
   Partial indices as depictors of periodontal disease status and treatment needs. J. Dent. Res., 1982, 61: 221 (Abstract).

5. *Ainamo J., Barmes D., Beagrie G., Cutress T., Martin J.* and *Sardo-Infirri J.*
   Development of the World Health Organization (WHO) Community Periodontal Index of Treatment Needs (CPITN). Int. Dent. J., 1982, 32: 281–291.

6. *Ainamo J.* and *Bay I.*
   Problems and proposals for recording gingivitis and plaque. Int. Dent. J., 1975, 25: 229–235.

7. *Axelsson P.* and *Lindhe J.*
   The significance of maintenance care in the treatment of periodontal disease. J. Clin. Periodontol., 1981, 8: 281–294.

8. *Baume L. J.*
   Limitations of simplified indices in prevalence studies of periodontal diseases. A survey of the school population of French Polynesia. Int. Dent. J., 1968, 18: 570–585.

9. *Bellini H. T.* and *Gjermo P.*
   Application of the Periodontal Treatment Need System (PTNS) in a group of Norwegian industrial employees. Community Dent. Oral Epidemiol. 1973, 1: 22–29.

10. *Brady W. F.* and *Martinoff J. T.*
    A simplified examination, diagnosis, and treatment classification of periodontal disease. J. Amer. Dent. Assoc., 1982, 104: 313–317.

11. *Carranza Jr., F. A.* (ed.)
    Glickman's Clinical Periodontology. Philadelphia: W. B. Saunders, 1979, pp. 319–351.

12. *Davies E. E., Ray H. G.* and *Fraleigh C. M.*
    A study of the need for periodontal treatment in a group of naval personnel with a comparison of periodontal indices. J. Amer. Dent. Assoc., 1961, 63: 503–512.

13. *Davies G. N.*
    Dental conditions among the Polynesians of Pukapuka (Danger Island). II. The prevalence of periodontal disease. J. Dent. Res., 1956, 35: 734–741.

14. *Davies G. N.*
    The different requirements of periodontal indices for prevalence studies and clinical trials. Int. Dent. J., 1968, 18: 560–569.

15. *Davies G. N., Kruger B. J.* and *Homan B. T.*
    An epidemiological training course. Aust. Dent. J., 1967, 12: 17–28.

16. *Ekanayaka A. N. I.*
    An Assessment of the Value of Indices in Quantifying Treatment Needs in Periodontal Disease. Ph. D. Thesis, University of London, 1976.

17. *Ekanayaka A. N. I.* and *Sheiham A.*
Estimating the time and personnel required to treat periodontal disease. J. Clin. Periodontol., 1978, 5: 85–94.

18. *Ekanayaka A. N. I.* and *Sheiham A.*
Assessing the periodontal treatment needs of a population. J. Clin. Periodontol., 1979, 6: 150–157.

19. *Greene J. C.*
Oral hygiene and periodontal disease. Amer. J. Public Health, 1963, 53: 913–922.

20. *Greene J. C.* and *Vermillion J. R.*
The Oral Hygiene Index: A method for classifying oral hygiene status. J. Amer. Dent. Assoc., 1960, 61: 172–179.

21. *Greene J. C.* and *Vermillion J. R.*
The simplified oral hygiene index. J. Amer. Dent. Assoc., 1964, 68: 7–13.

22. *Hansen F. R.* and *Johansen J. R.*
Periodontal treatment needs in 35-year-old citizens in Oslo. J. Clin. Periodontol., 1977, 4: 263–271.

23. *Jamison H. C.*
Prevalence and Severity of Periodontal Disease in a Sample of a Population. Ph. D. Thesis, University of Michigan, 1960.

24. *Jamison H. C.*
Some comparisons of two methods of assessing periodontal disease. Amer. J. Public Health, 1963, 53: 1102–1106.

25. *Johansen J. R., Gjermo P.* and *Bellini H. T.*
A system to classify the need for periodontal treatment. Acta Odontol. Scand., 1973, 31: 297–305.

26. *Kelly J. E.* and *Van Kirk C. E.*
Periodontal Disease in Adults, United States 1960-62. Washington, D. C., USPHS., U.S. Department of Health, Education and Welfare, National Center for Health Statistics, Publication No. 1000, Series 11, No. 12, 1966.

27. *Kjome R. L.*
Effects of Tooth Sample Selection on the Periodontal Disease Index. Ph. D. Thesis, University of Michigan, 1975.

28. *Lilienthal B., Amarena V.* and *Gregory G.*
A comparison of a modified periodontal scoring system with Russel's Periodontal Index. Arch. Oral Biol., 1964, 9: 575–583.

29. *Lindhe J., Hamp S. E.* and *Löe H.*
Plaque induced periodontal disease in Beagle dogs. J. Periodontal Res., 1975, 10: 243–255.

30. *Löe H.*
Epidemiology of periodontal disease. Odont. Tidskr., 1963, 71: 479–503.

31. *Löe H.*
The Gingival Index, the Plaque Index and the Retention Index systems. J. Periodontol., 1967, 38: 610–616.

32. *Löe H., Theilade E.* and *Jensen S. B.*
Experimental gingivitis in man. J. Periodontol., 1965, 36: 177–187.

33. *Lövdal A., Arno A., Schei O.* and *Waerhaug J.*
Combined effect of subgingival scaling and controlled oral hygiene on the incidence of gingivitis. Acta Odontol. Scand., 1961, 19: 537–555.

34. *Marthaler T. M., Engelberger B.* and *Rateitschak K. H.*
Bone loss in Ramfjord's index: substitution of selected teeth. Helv. Odontol. Acta, 1971, 15: 121–126.

35. *Mühlemann H. R.* and *Son S.*
Gingival Sulcus Bleeding – a leading symptom in initial gingivitis. Helv. Odontol. Acta, 1971 15: 105–113.

36. *O'Leary T. J.*
A study of periodontal examination systems. J. Dent. Res., 1964, 43: 794 (Abstract).

37. *O'Leary T. J.*
The periodontal screening examination. J. Periodontol., 1967 38: 617–624.

38. *O'Leary T. J., Gibson W. A., Shannon I. L., Schuessler C. F.* and *Nabers C. L.*
A screening examination for detection of gingival and periodontal breakdown and local irritants. Periodontics, 1963, 1: 167–174.

39. *Oliver R. C.*
Patient evaluation. Int. Dent. J., 1977, 27: 103–106.

40. *Quigley G.* and *Hein J. W.*
Comparative cleansing efficiency of manual and power brushing. J. Amer. Dent. Assoc., 1962, 65: 26–29.

41. *Ramfjord S. P.*
Indices for prevalence and incidence of periodontal disease. J. Periodontol., 1959, 30: 51–59.

42. *Ramfjord S. P.*
Methodology for determining periodontal treatment needs. J. Periodontol., 1969, 40: 524–528.

43. *Ramfjord S. D., Knowles J. W., Nissle R. R., Burgett F. G.* and *Shick R. A.*
Results following three modalities of periodontal therapy. J. Periodontol., 1975, 46: 522–526.

44. *Rosling B., Nyman S., Lindhe J.* and *Jern B.*
The healing potential of the periodontal tissues following different techniques of periodontal surgery in plaque-free dentitions. A 2 year clinical study. J. Clin. Periodontol., 1976, 3: 233–250.

45. *Russell A. L.*
A system of classification and scoring for prevalence surveys of periodontal disease. J. Dent. Res., 1956, 35: 350–359.

46. *Sandler H. C.* and *Stahl S.*
Measurement of periodontal disease prevalence. J. Amer. Dent. Assoc., 1959, 58: 93–97.

47. *Scherp H. W.*
Current concepts in periodontal research: epidemiological contributions. J. Amer. Dent. Assoc., 1964, 68: 667–675.

48. *Sheiham A.* and *Striffler D. F.*
A comparison of four epidemiological methods of assessing periodontal disease. I. Population findings. J. Periodontal Res., 1970, 5: 148–154.

49. *Sheiham A.* and *Striffler D. F.*
A comparison of four epidemiological methods of assessing periodontal disease. II. Test of periodontal indices. J. Periodontal Res., 1970, 5: 155–161.

50. *Silness J.* and *Löe H.*
Periodontal disease in pregnancy. II. Correlation between oral hygiene and periodontal condition. Acta Odontol. Scand., 1964, 22: 121–135.

51. *Waerhaug J.*
Epidemiology of periodontal disease. In Workshop in Periodontics (Ramfjord, Kerr and Ash eds.), Ann Arbor, Michigan, 1966, pp 179–211.

52. *Waerhaug J.*
Prevalence of periodontal disease in Ceylon. Association with age, sex, oral hygiene, socio-economic factors, vitamin deficiences, malnutrition, betel and tobacco consumption and ethnic group. Acta Odontol. Scand., 1967, 25: 205–231.

53. *WHO.*
Epidemiology, Etiology and Prevention of Periodontal Diseases. Technical Report Series 621, Geneva, 1978.

3. Prevalence of Periodontal Disease and Need for Periodontal Treatment in a Representative Sample of 35–44-year-olds in Copenhagen

John Christensen, Mogens R. Skougaard and Kaj Stoltze

Introduction

The prevalence of periodontal disease in the adult population of the western world is close to 100%[17, 22] and tooth mortality in adults is due at least as much to periodontal disease as to caries.[5, 9] Nevertheless only a small fraction of the effort of the dental services is aimed at the prevention and treatment of periodontal disease.[3] In recent years attempts have been made in the Scandinavian countries to change this pattern and it is encouraging that as of 1982 periodontal treatment is included in the agreement between the Danish National Health Service and the Dental Association.

The majority of investigations on periodontal conditions have been performed on more or less selected groups, mainly industrial employees.[3, 11, 12, 13, 14, 19] Examples of investigations dealing with randomly selected samples of total populations include those of *Håkansson*[7] and the large scale International Collaborative Study by the World Health Organization (WHO).[2] However, the final results of the WHO have not yet been published.

In recent years attempts have been made not only to describe the pattern of periodontal health, but also to evaluate the need for periodontal treatment in order to allow an estimate to be made of the resources, including dental manpower, necessary to achieve a significant improvement in periodontal health. *Johansen,*

Gjermo and *Bellini*[10] suggested a Periodontal Treatment Need System (PTNS) which assessed the need for treatment in each quadrant. The classification was based on criteria related to the state of periodontal health of the quadrant in question. PTNS has been used in a number of investigations, often in slightly modified versions.[3, 6, 12]

The purpose of the present investigation was to determine the prevalence and severity of periodontal disease and assess the need for periodontal treatment in a representative sample of 35–44-year-olds in Copenhagen and to estimate the time required for adequate periodontal treatment of the total population expressed in dental man-hours.

Material and Method
Study sample

The study sample comprised 400 persons drawn from Denmark's computerized Central Population Registry (CPR). CPR contains demographic data on all permanent residents in Denmark.

The sample was selected at random from 35–44-year-olds living in the Copenhagen and Frederiksberg municipalities. Geographically, Frederiksberg lies within Copenhagen but has the status of an independent municipality. There are no suburban areas within either of the municipalities.

The 400 persons selected represented 0.7% of the total population of 35–44-year-olds in Copenhagen and Frederiksberg. Those who had died or moved from the area during the interval between the selection and the actual start of the investigation were deleted from the sample because these individuals had not been informed of the investigation and could not therefore be classified as non-responders.

Procedure

Permission was granted by the Danish Ministry of the Interior for the following information to be released from the CPR:

1. Name.
2. CPR-number.
3. Address.
4. Marital status.
5. Occupation.

The following procedures were carried out for the study:

1. Letter of introduction

A letter of introduction was mailed to all participants. The letter gave information on the scope of the study and advised the participants that they would be contacted by a public health nurse for an interview and an appointment for a subsequent home visit by a dentist for dental examination.

2. Interview by public health nurse

The public health nurses have considerable experience in gaining access to private homes for health care purposes and could therefore be expected to reduce the non-response rate.

The purpose of the interview was to obtain unbiased information from the subjects on frequency of dental visits, previous participation in the school dental service, and on their own opinion of their need for periodontal treatment.

3. Dental examination

Following the appointment made by the public health nurse, the dental investigator (JC) performed the dental examinations in the homes of the subjects. The interviews, as well as the dental examinations, were conducted in the evenings and at weekends in order to minimize the non-response rate.

Examination methods

Portable equipment was used for the examination including fibre optic light, disposable mirrors and standardized graduated periodontal probes.

The periodontium of each subject was examined using a modified version of the Periodontal Treatment Need System (PTNS).[10] According to PTNS, each quadrant is scored in one of the following categories:

Class 0 – no treatment needed.
Class A – motivation and oral hygiene instruction.
Class B – scaling and removal of overhangs.
Class C – surgery

The modifications applied were as follows:

All teeth were scored after an examination of all surfaces in order to obtain detailed information on the periodontal health status of each subject and data which could be used as a baseline for a longitudinal study. Scoring of quadrants was performed by computer, the overall score for each quadrant being that of the worst tooth in the quadrant in accordance with the original index.

A score of D was assigned for teeth with

Table 3.1 Distribution of the 319 responders by socio-economic status and sex.

Socioeconomic status	Females		Males		Total	
	Number	%	Number	%	Number	%
Low	67	41.3	47	29.9	114	35.7
Middle	85	52.5	85	54.2	170	53.3
High	10	6.2	25	15.9	35	11.0
Total	162	100.0	157	100.0	319	100.0

advanced destruction of the supporting tissues and loss of masticatory function.

A quadrant was not given the score C, if C was assigned it was only to the last tooth in the dental arch or to a tooth with no neighbouring teeth.

The last modification was introduced in order to avoid an overestimation of the time required for treatment of a single tooth, for example, a tooth in contact with a partial denture.

The examiner was calibrated with a trained periodontal epidemiologist and intra-examiner variability was calculated from replicate examination of 20 patients. The reproducibility was found to be 90%.

The data were analysed statistically by computer using the 'Statistical Analysis System' (SAS).[18]

Results

Of the 400 subjects originally drawn from CPR, 42 were excluded. One of these had died, 27 had moved away from the greater Copenhagen area, and 14 were incorrectly listed by CPR. Thus the actual sample was reduced to 358. Five subjects were interviewed but refused a dental examination, 22 refused to participate in the interview or the dental examination, and 12 were unwilling to participate for various other stated reasons, such as illness. The overall response rate was 89%.

The subjects were classified socioeconomically on the basis of their occupation, as described by *Antoft* and *Jensen*.[1] However, for the present study the number of social groups was reduced to 3, viz. low, middle and high. The distribution of the responders by sex and socioeconomic status is shown in Table 1.

Number of teeth

Twenty-five, or 7.8%, of the 319 subjects examined were edentulous. Edentulousness was more frequent among women (9.3%) than among men (6.4%). The difference was, however, not statistically significant ($x^2 = 0,92$, df = 1, $0.30 < P < 0.40$). The prevalence of dentate subjects without teeth in the upper jaw was approximately the same as that of subjects edentulous. The prevalence of edentulousness was closely related to socio-economic status, the rate being almost three times higher in the low than in the high socio-economic group.

The dentate portion of the study sample comprised 294 subjects, and the analyses which follow were performed on this part of the sample. Table 3.2 shows the num-

Table 3.2 Number of teeth in the 294 dentate by sex.

	Number	1 – 9 teeth		10 – 19 teeth		20 or more teeth	
		Number	%	Number	%	Number	%
Women	147	14	9.5	21	14.3	112	76.2
Men	147	5	3.4	21	14.3	121	82.3
Total	294	19	6.5	42	14.3	233	79.3

Table 3.3 PTNS scores in the 294 dentate subjects according to tooth number. (No. 1. Central incisors, No. 8: Third molars).

	Tooth Number	1	2	3	4	5	6	7	8
PTNS	0	12.1	10.2	9.7	7.7	5.8	4.8	3.0	0.0
score	A	10.1	12.0	11.6	9.1	10.1	4.8	6.1	3.3
%	B	62.1	65.5	61.3	62.6	69.2	73.1	66.6	60.8
	C	15.2	12.0	17.4	20.1	14.2	17.3	24.3	35.8
	D	0.6	0.2	0.0	0.5	0.7	0.0	0.0	0.0
	C + D	15.8	12.2	17.4	20.6	14.9	17.3	24.3	35.8
PTNS	0	1.2	2.3	4.0	3.1	4.4	3.8	3.9	1.2
score	A	0.5	1.2	1.9	4.2	3.6	6.0	2.3	1.2
%	B	90.4	88.7	81.7	77.9	75.4	74.0	67.5	44.1
	C	6.7	8.1	12.2	14.8	16.5	16.0	26.0	53.4
	D	1.1	0.7	0.2	0.0	0.0	0.0	0.2	0.0
	C + D	7.8	8.8	12.4	14.8	16.5	16.0	26.2	53.4

ber of teeth in men and women, and indicates that the men had slightly more standing teeth. However, the difference was not statistically significant ($x^2 = 4.61$, df = 2, $0.05 < P < 0.10$).

The theoretical number of quadrants in the 294 dentate subjects was 1176, though as a result of missing teeth the number was reduced to 1068 according to the guidelines described in PTNS.

Periodontal status

PTNS is designed primarily for the purpose of estimating treatment need. The PTNS criteria, however, are described in terms of symptoms of the disease as well as in terms of appropriate treatment.

Table 3.3 shows the percentage distribution of the PTNS scores for the teeth in the upper and lower jaw. It is evident that score B was predominant with between 61% and 90% of the teeth receiving this score (gingivitis and calculus).

Score C, indicating pockets of 5 mm depth and more, varied from 7% to 53%; when the 3rd molars were excluded the latter figure was reduced to 26%. The prevalence of sound teeth was highest in the upper anterior sextant, but was low in the anterior sextant of the lower jaw. The overall percentage of sound teeth was only 4.8%. The prevalence of gingivitis without calculus formation (score A) was low. Among the lower front teeth only 0.8% were given this score.

The PTNS values, quoted so far, have been registered according to the original criteria described by *Johansen et al,*[10] with the exception that each individual tooth was scored. When used in this manner, PTNS is closely similar to *Russell's* Periodontal Index (PI).[16] In order to facilitate comparison to other studies, the PTNS scores were transformed into PI as follows:

PTNS	PI
0	0
A	1
B	2
C	6
D	8

It was apparent that for each individual tooth scores, transformed in terms of PI, the PI was systematically higher in men than in women, and in both jaws the lowest PI values were found in the incisors. The mean PI score for the two jaws by sex are shown in Table 3.4. The overall PI mean for the study sample was 2.5.

Table 3.4 Mean PI sex calculated from the PTNS scores (Third molars not included).

	Upper jaw	Lower jaw	Both jaws
Female	2.17	2.23	2.20
Male	2.72	2.73	2.72
Total	2.45	2.48	2.46

In Table 3.5 the 294 subjects are listed according to highest PTNS score and sex. Only two persons, or 0.7%, had a completely healthy periodontium. None had gingivitis in the absence of calculus, 57% had gingivitis and calculus but without pocket formation, whereas 37% had pockets in at least one quadrant. The number of men with scores C and D was significantly higher than women ($x^2 = 8.74$, df = 1, $0.001 < P < 0.005$). These and the following figures were based on the modified PTNS described on page 48.

In Table 3.6 the 1068 quadrants are listed according to PTNS score and sex. This more detailed analysis of the periodontal picture shows that the frequency of quadrants given score A was about the

Table 3.5 The 294 dentate subjects listed by sex and maximum PTNS score.

		Maximum Score					
		Female		Male		Female + Male	
		Number	%	Number	%	Number	%
Score 0		2	1.36	0	0.00	2	0.70
	A	0	0.00	0	0.00	0	0.00
	B	96	65.31	73	49.66	169	57.48
	C	46	31.29	64	43.54	110	37.42
	D	3	2.04	10	6.80	13	4.40
	C + D	49	33.33	74	50.34	123	41.81
Total		147	100.00	147	100.00	294	100.00

Table 3.6 The 1068 quadrants in the dentate subjects listed according to PTNS score and sex.

	Number of Quadrants					
	Female		Male		Female + Male	
	Number	%	Number	%	Number	%
Score 0	12	2.29	0	0.00	12	1.12
A	10	1.91	1	0.18	11	1.03
B	394	75.19	362	66.54	756	70.79
C	105	20.04	169	31.07	274	25.66
D	3	0.57	12	2.21	15	1.40
C + D	108	20.61	181	33.28	289	27.06
Total	524	100.00	544	100.00	1068	100.00

Table 3.7 The 1068 quadrants in the dentate subjects listed according to PTNS score and socio-economic status.

	Number of Quadrants					
	Low		Middle		High	
	Number	%	Number	%	Number	%
Score 0	6	1.81	6	0.99	0	0.00
A	2	0.61	8	1.32	1	0.76
B	224	67.67	433	71.57	99	75.00
C	93	28.10	149	24.63	32	24.24
D	6	1.81	9	1.49	0	0.00
C + D	99	29.91	158	26.12	32	24.24
Total	331	100.00	605	100.00	132	100.00

same as that given score 0 (1%). Furthermore Table 3.6 confirms the earlier observation that males had more severe periodontal disease than females. The prevalence of quadrants with C and D scores was significantly higher in men than in women ($x^2 = 21.67$ df = 1, P<0.0005).
In Table 3.7 the PTNS scores for the quadrants are related to socio-economic status. Only slight differences were observed which were not statistically significant ($x^2 = 2.17$, df = 2, 030<P <0.40). An analysis of the PTNS scores related to the marital status also revealed no significant differences.
Fifty-nine per cent of the 294 subjects saw a dentist regularly, i.e. at least once a year. It can be seen from Table 3.8 that the number of subjects with the maximum score C and D was highest among the irregular attenders ($x^2 = 27.14$, df = 1, P<0.0005). Sixty per cent of the subjects

Table 3.8 Number of quadrants by score related to whether or not the subjects visited the dentist regularly.

		Regular		Nonregular	
		Number of quadrants		Number of quadrants	
		Number	%	Number	%
Score	0	12	1.8	0	0.0
	A	10	1.5	1	0.2
	B	449	75.2	257	63.6
	C	141	21.2	133	32.9
	D	2	0.3	13	3.2
	C + D	143	21.5	146	36.1
Total		664	100.0	404	100.0

Table 3.9 Maximum PTNS score and number of quadrants by score related to whether or not the subjects had received periodontal treatment.

		Previous periodontal treatment				No periodontal treatment			
		Maximum Score		Number of quadrants		Maximum Score		Number of quadrants	
		Number	%	Number	%	Number	%	Number	%
Score	0	1	1.4	4	1.6	1	0.4	8	1.0
	A	0	0.0	5	1.9	0	0.0	6	0.7
	B	29	41.4	147	57.0	140	62.5	609	75.2
	C	37	52.9	98	38.0	73	32.6	176	21.7
	D	3	4.3	4	1.6	10	4.5	11	1.4
	C + D	40	57.2	102	39.6	83	37.1	187	23.1
Total		70	100.0	258	100.0	224	100.0	810	100.0

had participated in regular school dental care programmes as children. The PTNS scores of these persons did not differ from those who had not attended the school dental service.

About 25% of the subjects had undergone periodontal treatment. Thirty-one per cent of these stated that they had been given instruction and motivation in oral hygiene, 23% had had scaling for periodontal purposes, 31% had undergone periodontal surgery, and 47% had been subject to other periodontal treatment.

In Table 3.9 the dentate part of the study sample is listed according to highest score, and grouped according to whether or not the subjects had received periodontal treatment. Table 3.9 also shows the distribution of quadrants by score in the two groups and it can be seen that the prevalence of maximum score C and D was higher among those who had been

53

treated for periodontal conditions. This difference was highly significant ($x = 8.82$, df $= 1$, $0.001 < P < 0.005$). The number of score C and D quadrants was also higher in the treated group. ($x^2 = 26.81$, df $= 2$, $P < 0.0005$).

During the interview the subjects were asked whether they considered that they had gingivitis or periodontal disease. An analysis of the questionnaire data revealed that the individuals who stated that they had received periodontal treatment were almost all the same ones who were aware of having periodontal disease.

Periodontal treatment need

Johansen et al.[10] have estimated the time requirements per quadrant for the treatment of the PTNS classes A, B and C. According to this estimate, score A requires 60 minutes per patient, score B needs 30 minutes, and score C needs 60 minutes per quadrant. If these figures were applied to the present observations, the treatment times outlined in Table 3.10 would be required.

In addition to 652 hours, 292 persons would need class A treatment, i.e. individual oral hygiene motivation and instruction. Thus the total time requirement for the periodontal treatment of the 294 dentate subjects would be 944 hours.

Table 3.10 Treatment times.

	Number of quadrants	Hours
Score B	756	378
Score C	274	274
Total	1030	652

Discussion

One of the problems related to examining randomly selected samples is that it often proves difficult to obtain a high response rate.[19] In the present study this was close to 90%, which can be regarded as satisfactory.

The fact that the index was applied to each tooth increased the validity of the PTNS index in the assessment of periodontal health status. The findings in the present study were by and large in agreement with those from other periodontal surveys, viz. a high prevalence of gingivitis and loss of attachment.

The percentage of edentulous individuals was lower than the percentage in the same age group examined by *Plasschaert et al*[14] in the Netherlands. It is noteworthy that the Dutch investigation reported twice as many edentulous men as women, whereas the present investigation revealed 1.5 times as many woman as men. The number of teeth in the dentate population was slightly higher in the Dutch study sample. The positive correlation between educational level and the number of teeth in that study was the same as that found between socio-economic status and number of teeth in the present study. The results of the periodontal examination showed that the prevalence of gingivitis with calculus formation among the 35–44 year olds was high in both studies.

In the Danish replicate of the International Collaborative Study (ICS) which was carried out in Århus, the mean PI for this age group was found to be 2.0.[4] The fact that this figure is lower than that found in the present study probably reflects the dissimilarity between the two scoring systems since the clinical examinations were carried out by the same person (JC). The main difference is probably not so much due to differences between PI and PTNS, provided the latter is scored for each tooth. The most likely explanation is rather that in the WHO study the periodontal probe was used only on teeth where pathological pocket formation was suspected from visual inspection, whereas in the present study every tooth was probed on all surfaces. In the Norwegian part of ICS, the mean PI was 1.3,[23] which is considerably lower than the Danish PI values. Even if interexaminer variability accounted for some of the difference, the figures seem to indicate a somewhat better periodontal health status among the 35–44 year olds in Norway than in Denmark.

Sheiham[19] found mean PI values of 4.3 among 35–44 year olds in England, a 72% higher level than that found in the present study. This is consistent with the difference in the prevalence rates of periodontal pockets found in the two studies. In Britain, 97% of the age group had pocketing compared to 37% with PTNS score C in the present investigation. Interexaminer variability and the use of slightly different scoring systems may account in part for these dissimilarities. Nevertheless, the results seem to indicate a higher prevalence of severe periodontal conditions in Britain than in Denmark.

With regard to the prevalence of pocket formation, our results are in agreement with those reported by Håkansson[7] and by Bellini and Gjermo.[3] Both these studies reported 40% pocketing among the age group in question.

The relationship between socio-economic, or educational levels, and the prevalence of pocket formation appears to be somewhat obscure. In the present study only slight differences occurred between the three socio-economic groups. This observation is in agreement with the results reported by Sheiham[19] and Bellini and Gjermo,[3] whereas Plasschaert et al[14] found decreasing prevalence of pocket formation with increasing level of education. Petersen[13] examined employees from a Danish industrial firm and found the prevalence of sound teeth was significantly greater among the high than among the low income groups. Furthermore, the

prevalence of PTNS score C in the highest income group was only 40% of that found in the lowest income group. The evaluation of differences in periodontal health in relation to socio-economic status, however, is complicated by the fact that the lower income groups have fewer teeth than the middle and high income groups.

It was revealed from the interviews that 60% of the subjects saw a dentist once a year or more. This figure is in agreement with the findings of Jensen[8] and Schwarz and Hansen,[20] who analysed dental visiting habits in Danish urban areas, and with those of Håkansson[7] from Sweden.

The present study demonstrates that more than 99% of the study sample had gingivitis with calculus or pocket formation regardless of the frequency of dental visiting. However, the prevalence of pocket formation was lower among those who visited the dentist regularly than among those who did not. The difference was emphasized by the fact that regular visitors had more teeth than the non-regular. The difference may be due to better oral hygiene among the regular group. The PTNS does not yield any information on the amount of calculus present though it seems reasonable to assume that regular dental visitors would have less calculus than irregular. Nevertheless, it is noteworthy that calculus was found on practically all subjects who saw the dentist at least once a year.

The 70 persons who stated that they had been treated for periodontal disease had a higher prevalence of pocketing than the rest of the sample. It is reasonable to assume that those who had been treated for periodontal disease had a poorer periodontal condition before the treatment than the rest of the group. On the other hand, it is difficult to maintain too optimistic a view on the effect of the periodontal treatment of this group considering the high prevalence of gingivitis with calculus and with pocket formation. The interviews did not reveal an awareness of periodontal problems among the study sample. The persons who stated that they had periodontal disease were the same as those who had received periodontal treatment. Therefore, it was not possible to distinguish between the ones who had been treated on their own initiative and those who had been informed of their periodontal problems by the dentist.

The time required for periodontal treatment of the sample was estimated at 944 hours, according to PTNS. This estimate is somewhat lower than that made by *Bellini* and *Gjermo*,[3] who assessed the time required for periodontal treatment of 313 dentate subjects as 1292 hours, corresponding to 1214 hours for 294 persons. The PTNS described by *Johansen et al*[10] results in a higher number of quadrants with a score of C than the modified version of the index used in the present study. A recalculation in accordance with the original PTNS criteria shifted the distribution of quadrants given the scores B and C, resulting in an increase of 37 hours treatment time for the 294 subjects. The remaining difference of 233 hours between the present study and that by *Bellini* and *Gjermo*[3] is probably due to the fact that the Norwegian sample comprised all age groups. This confirms the observation that treatment need increases when older age groups are included.[3, 14, 19]

The total population of 35–44 year olds in Copenhagen and Frederiksberg municipalities is approximately 60000; hence the time required for their periodontal treatment would be around 180000 hours, while approximately 1750000 hours would be required for the country's total population in this age group. This estimate is of course extremely crude, and even more so if an attempt is made to assess the order of magnitude of the treatment need for the entire population between 25 and 65 years of age. If a bold extrapolation is made, the total need for periodontal treatment of the adult population in Denmark

would require around 7.5 million treatment hours or one year's fulltime work for all the 5000 dentists in Denmark. Although somewhat higher, this assessment is comparable to the estimate made by *Sheiham* and *Smales*[20] in the UK. According to *Sheiham* and *Smales* the need for periodontal treatment of the adult British population would require the work of all the dentists in the country for 160 days per year. Even when the allowance is made for the crudeness of these assessments, the order of magnitude of the figures demonstrates that periodontal disease cannot be eliminated through traditional treatment.

Periodontal conditions are not likely to be significantly improved unless the main emphasis is placed on preventive measures, primarily aimed at changing oral hygiene behaviour through systematic health education. A realistic approach could be the involvement of dental auxiliaries to a much greater extent in preventive activities and simpler types of treatment.

References

1. *Antoft P.* and *Jensen K.*
   Socialklasseinddeling ved hjælp af stillings-betegnelse. Tandlægebladet, 1976, 80: 187–193.

2. *Barmes D. E.*
   A progress report on adult data analysis in the WHO/USPHS International Collaborative Study. Int. Dent. J., 1978, 28: 348–364.

3. *Bellini H. T.* and *Gjermo P.*
   Application of the Periodontal Treatment Need System (PTNS) in a group of Norwegian industrial employees. Community Dent. Oral Epidemiol., 1973, 1: 22–29.

4. *Christensen J.*
   Replicate of the International Collaborative Study carried out in Århus, Denmark, 1982 (Unpublished manuscript.)

5. *Gad T.* and *Bay I.*
   Årsagen til tandekstraktioner af permanente tænder i Danmark. Tandlægebladet, 1972, 76: 103–114.

6. *Helöe L. A.*
Oral health status and treatment needs in a disadvantaged rural population in Norway. Community Dent. Oral Epidemiol., 1973, 1: 94–103.

7. *Håkansson J.*
Dental care habits, attitudes towards dental health and dental status among 20–60 year old individuals in Sweden. Thesis, Malmø, 1978.

8. *Jensen K.*
Dental care practices and socio-economic status in Denmark. Community Dent. Oral Epidemiol., 1974, 2: 273–281.

9. *Johansen J. R.*
A survey in Norway for causes of loss of permanent teeth and the number of teeth remaining after extraction. Thesis, Oslo, 1970.

10. *Johansen J. R.*, *Gjermo P.* and *Bellini H. T.*
A system to classify the need for periodontal treatment. Acta Odontol. Scand., 1973, 31: 297–305.

11. *Lövdal A.*, *Arno A.* and *Waerhaug J.*
Incidence of clinical manifestations of periodontal disease in light of oral hygiene and calculus formation. J. Amer. Dent. Assoc., 1958, 56: 21–33.

12. *Markanen H.*
Periodontal treatment need in a Finnish industrial population. Community Dent. Oral Epidemiol., 1978, 6: 240–244.

13. *Petersen P. E.*
Tandplejeadfærd, tandstatus samt odontologisk behandlingsbehov blandt arbejdere og funktionærer på en stor dansk industrivirksomhed. En socialodontologisk bedriftsundersøgelse. Thesis, Copenhagen, 1981.

14. *Plasschaert A. J. M.*, *Folmer T.*, *van den Heuvel J. L. M.*, *Jansen J.*, *van Opijnen L.* and *Wouters S. L. J.*
An epidemiologic survey of periodontal disease in Dutch adults. Community Dent. Oral Epidemiol., 1978, 4: 221–226.

15. *Richards A. D.*, *Willcocks A. J.*, *Bulman J. S.* and *Slack G. L.*
A survey of the dental health and attitudes towards dentistry in two communities. Part 1 sociological data. Brit. Dent. J., 1965, 118: 199–205.

16. *Russell A. L.*
A system of classification and scoring for prevalence surveys of periodontal disease. J. Dent. Res., 1956, 35: 350–359.

17. *Russell A. L.*
Periodontal disease incidence in the United States. In The Periodontal Needs of the United States Population: Workshop Report. (O'Leary, T. J., ed.) Chicago, 1967, pp. 28–35.

18. SAS: Statistical Analysis System. SAS Institute Inc., North Carolina 1982.

19. *Sheiham A.*
The prevalence and severity of periodontal disease in British populations. Brit. Dent. J., 1969, 126: 115–122.

20. *Sheiham A.* and *Smales F. C.*
Suggestions for Improving Dental Health and Dental Services. Dental evidence submitted to the Royal Commission on the National Health Service, 1977.

21. *Schwarz E.* and *Randers Hansen E.*
Utilization of dental services in the adult Danish population 1975. Community Dent. Oral Epidemiol., 1976, 4: 221–226.

22. *Waerhaug J.*
Epidemiology of periodontal disease. Review of literature. In: World Workshop in Periodontics. (Ramfjord S. P., Kerr D. A. and Ash M. M. eds.) Ann Arbor 1966, p. 179–211.

23. WHO: International Collaborative Study of Dental Manpower Systems. Interim report, Geneva, 1979.

4. An Analysis of Existing Dental Services in Relation to Periodontal Care

Aubrey Sheiham

Introduction

Chronic periodontal diseases are very common in all European countries and are frequently cited as the major cause of tooth loss in adults. The reason for the persistence of periodontal diseases, despite the availability of favourable numbers of dental personnel in some areas, is considered to be due to one or more of the following:

1. The failure of dentists to diagnose and treat the disease.
2. The ineffectiveness of the treatments.
3. The inappropriateness and ineffectiveness of the health education instructions given.
4. The poor oral health care motivation of the public.
5. The limited role of dental personnel in controlling periodontal diseases.

Before analysing the reasons for the limitations of the existing dental services to control periodontal disease, the implicit goal – that all levels of periodontal disease should be eliminated needs to be questioned. Periodontal health is considered to be the absence of gingivitis, no loss of attachment and anatomically perfect gingival contours; the absence of disease or its consequences. However, there is still controversy among histologists and pathologists about the definition of normal periodontal tissues. The Committee on Structure and Metabolism of the Normal Periodontium at the International Conference on Research in the Biology of Periodontal Disease[3] recognized that '... there was a gradient rather than a sharp line in separating health from disease'. In addition, there is doubt about what forms of gingivitis are 'contained' gingivitis and which will develop into periodontitis.[23] Very few gingival lesions do progress and many regress.[21]. In addition to gingivitis remaining contained to the gingivae, periodontal pockets can remain unchanged for considerable periods and frequently regress[21] with reformation of alveolar bone[16] without treatment. These features of periodontal disease suggest that the dominant model of chronic periodontal disease – gingivitis progressing invariably to periodontitis which is progressively destructive – is not the only model of the disease. Some lesions stay contained for long periods. Others remain quiescent for long periods and then progress either slowly or rapidly. *MacPhee* and *Muir*[12] have suggested that 'In some individuals at some point in time this stable lesion becomes converted into a slowly progressively destructive lesion for reasons which are not presently clear'. While the evidence suggests that 'contained' gingivitis is virtually the norm, particularly in the young individual, the probability is that the occurrence of the progressive lesion with increasing age is episodic and even well-established periodontitis may well have prolonged contained non-destructive phases.

If the rate of progression of periodontal

59

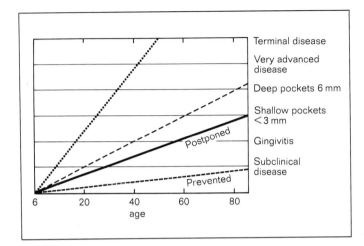

Terminal disease

Very advanced disease

Deep pockets 6 mm

Shallow pockets <3 mm

Gingivitis

Subclinical disease

Fig. 4.1 The possible clinical courses of chronic periodontal disease. An important strategy for controlling the disease is to alter the rate (slope) at which the disease develops thus postponing advanced disease or even preventing loss of periodontal attachment.

diseases is difficult to predict and the available epidemiological evidence indicates that the rate of progression is very slow in most people [11, 16, 20, 21] — 0.1 to 0.05 mm per year, the need to actively treat all people with periodontal disease is unjustified. Pilot,[13] in reviewing the ultimate objectives of dental care in relation to periodontal health, stated that it is the '... maintenance of a healthy natural functioning dentition throughout life, including all the social and biological functions as aesthetics, chewing, taste, speech, no discomfort, in the light of personal well-being of the individual'. This objective does not imply that all 32 teeth will have physiologically and anatomically perfect periodontal support with the attachment at the cemento-enamel junction. People do not die healthy. A certain level of structural change can be tolerated. In other words, some change in periodontal support is acceptable if that change does not affect the functioning of the dentition and is aesthetically acceptable to the person.

The patterns and rates of progression of periodontal disease differs from one individual to another. Many people have slow or zero rates of progression of disease. At the other extreme, a few have rapidly progressive disease. Others have intermediate rates (Fig. 4.1). It is known that more people will have a high rate of progression when the population has a high overall plaque score and a low rate when the plaque score is low.[11] But even within populations with overall low plaque scores, some groups have high scores and will therefore be at higher risk of more rapidly progressive periodontal disease which may lead to terminal disease by middle age.

Preventive and Treatment Strategies

A comprehensive plan for prevention has three components:

1. **A population strategy** for altering lifestyle and environmental characteristics, and their social and economic determinants;

2. **A high-risk strategy** for bringing preventive care to individuals at special risk;

3. **Secondary prevention** for averting or retarding progression of disease in those already affected and reducing recurrence.

The Population strategy

The population strategy is the most likely to benefit the periodontal status of the majority of people because: (1) a reduction in plaque scores in everybody will reduce the general rate of progression of disease and therefore many fewer teeth will be extracted than if efforts are concentrated on the small number of high-risk people. Indeed the WHO Scientific Group on Epidemiology, Etiology and Prevention of Periodontal Diseases[23] said that 'The dentist-patient approach to reducing tooth loss from periodontal disease is largely ineffective at a community level. Public health education and prevention must be undertaken to achieve the goals of keeping teeth for life and eliminating suffering, pain and loss of function from periodontal diseases. The need for such an approach has been demonstrated through the WHO international collaborative study on dental manpower systems. Unless an approach of this kind is adopted, all efforts at present expended on the repair and prevention of dental caries will be largely wasted'. (2) social pressure – although few dentists are optimistic about their ability to achieve satisfactory plaque control in their dental patients, and to maintain it, many people make strenuous efforts to clean their mouths because cleanliness is socially acceptable. So, in health education, the aim should be to create social pressure that makes healthy behaviour easier and more acceptable, thereby bringing social rewards for those who conform.

Many social and educational variables influence oral hygiene behaviour. The most important is sociopsychological variables such as socialization – the process whereby informed knowledge, values, attitudes and routines are transmitted to individuals through social interaction.[24] Young children copy the toothbrushing habits of their parents and teachers[1, 15].

In adolescents, toothbrushing is an integral part of personal hygiene and grooming behaviours which are influenced by the family and peers[8]. Because tooth cleaning is associated with grooming and personal hygiene, the majority of people do clean their teeth regularly. The objective of health education is to improve the effectiveness of oral hygiene behaviours. Since oral hygiene behaviour is part of general hygiene behaviour, programmes directed at improving oral cleanliness should be incorporated with health education directed at improving body hygiene and good grooming[18, 19]. Programmes should contain community leader education, public and mass media education, environmental change, and professional education.

Community leader education

This approach seeks to improve health behaviour through the better understanding and involvement of leaders of public opinion. Their serving as role models and their management skills help to implement preventive strategies.

Public education

This approach seeks to increase awareness and knowledge of good health behaviours by educating all age groups in a continuing, consistent programme. Direct education may include the following:

– education at work places, primary health care facilities such as ante-natal and well-women clinics combined with health information;
– adult education classes on prevention;
– school health programmes emphasizing teaching by peers of good health behaviours.

Mass media education

This approach seeks to increase community awareness of body hygiene and oral cleanliness, the availability of oral hygiene aids and plaque-disclosing agents to be used for feedback. Detailed information should be provided through written media-newspapers, magazines, pamphlets.

Environmental change

Encouragement of more healthy community behaviour may be achieved by modifying the environment. Examples of this are improvements in hygiene in the work place, provision of washing facilities, and the introduction of marketing practices promoting the use of oral hygiene aids.

Professional education

This approach aims to improve the oral hygiene instruction by professional personnel. Teachers, nursery school attendants, health visitors, nurses, doctors, dentists and other dental personnel and health educators should be provided with specific oral hygiene education so that they will provide accurate information and set good examples.

The High-Risk strategy

Dentists are trained to feel responsible for patients and, from that position, accepting responsibility for those at high-risk of dental diseases is not too difficult a transition. If a person is found to have a high plaque score, poor oral hygiene habits, is poorly educated and comes from a poor household, that person can be considered to have a high-risk of developing progressive periodontal disease.

Screening surveys to detect individuals at high-risk of periodontal disease should use social as well as clinical measures. We know that a high percentage of people with debris scores above 1.0 will have a relatively rapid rate of progression of periodontal disease per year[18]. If they also have a number of adverse socio-dental in-dicators, which will increase their vulnerability, then they should be classified as high-risk and special efforts should be made to reduce the risk factors. Depending on the numbers of people in the high-risk group, the approaches to reducing the risk factors will vary. But whatever the numbers, the programme should use a variety of methods from individual instruction using feedback methods[6] to group methods incorporated into general health education programmes.

Secondary prevention

A substantial proportion of periodontitis exists in people already known to have the disease. Measures to influence the course of already recognized periodontitis will help to reduce the total tooth loss from periodontal disease.

The principal therapeutic strategy is to reduce the amount of plaque. The methods of persuading patients to improve their oral cleanliness have been reviewed elsewhere.[17, 18] The current methods used by dentists have major shortcomings. Among these shortcomings is the failure to recognise that the methods are more appropriate to acute diseases, which ensure a higher rate of short-term compliance, than to chronic diseases which require long-term behaviour change.

If patients think that the treatment will lead to permanent cure they will relapse to their former patterns of oral hygiene. In addition, the commonly used method of oral hygiene instruction is based on an incorrect learning theory for behaviour change – that knowledge is a prerequisite for attitude and behaviour change.[17, 18] Furthermore the frequent repetition and exhortations to improve oral hygiene may have a dampening effect on motivation for both the patients and educators, thus reducing any effect which may have been achieved.[7]

In addition to the shortcomings of the

most important aspect of periodontal therapy, i.e. plaque control, doubt exists about the most effective way to treat existing periodontitis. *Ramfjord*[14] has listed six dogmas which have been proven to be partially or completely wrong:

1. Clinically probeable treated or untreated periodontal pockets of more than 3 mm are progressively destructive lesions.
2. Gingivitis and recurrence of periodontitis with progressive loss of attachment is inevitable if the teeth are not kept plaque-free by the patient after periodontal treatment.
3. The gingiva and the bone around teeth with periodontal pockets have to be sculputured surgically to resemble horizontal alveolar atrophy to the level of the deepest pocket, otherwise the destructive disease will progress.
4. Teeth with furcation involvement have such a poor prognosis that they should be extracted unless the furcation involvement can be eliminated by odontoplasty or root sectioning.
5. The deeper the pockets are, the poorer the prognosis for the teeth.
6. In general, advanced periodontal disease cannot be stopped by treatment, but the inevitable tooth loss may be delayed by disease 'control'.

Sheiham[17] has questioned two other commonly held beliefs about treatment and found little evidence to support their use. These are that all hard deposits must be removed, leaving a smooth tooth surface, and that teeth should be professionally cleaned at six-monthly intervals.

From this review of the strategies, which can be adopted to achieve the objective of maintaining a functional aesthetically and socially acceptable natural dentition for the life-span of most people, it is apparent that a combination of the three strategies – a population strategy, a high-risk strategy and a secondary preventive one – is necessary. The balance of effort should be heavily weighted to the population and high-risk strategies. If these strategies are adopted, the need for treatment will be reduced and treatment will be more successful. Treatment of periodontal disease requires an integrated approach involving improved oral hygiene habit formation, reinforcement and encouragement, and assessment to check whether any loss of attachment is occurring and, if so, at what rate.

The person should be treated as a long term case with the main emphasis on reinforcing good oral hygiene behaviour. Instead, most dentists and dental services concentrate on mechanistic solutions such as scaling, root planing and surgery.

Current Systems of Dental Care

The approach to dental care which has come to dominate the dental health care systems in much of the developed world, can broadly be characterized by a number of separate but related trends:

1. An orientation towards treatment and attempted cure rather than prevention.
2. An increasingly technological approach to diagnosis and treatment.
3. Increasing specialization and fragmentation of care.

The dominant philosophy of modern dental care is based upon the engineering approach to the body and the germ theory of disease. The mouth is considered as a collection of parts to be rescued from the effects of malfunction or breakdown primarily by technical intervention. The dentist is seen as a technician who repairs and occasionally services the machine. This philosophy promotes the concept of how a society can make progress in health, namely, by investing in the greater and greater provision of highly technological treatment services. However, for a number of reasons, there are growing doubts whether such an approach can lead to progress in dental health. Indeed, it may undermine prevention by diverting resources away from prevention and by encouraging unnecessary treatments.

The major shortcomings of the current systems have been highlighted recently. Firstly, the International Collaborative Study[2] has provided very important insights into the strenghts and weaknesses of the dominant systems. Their most significant finding was that none of the systems studied was able to prevent a large number of teeth being extracted from people by the age of 35–44 years. The findings from this study highlight four important factors about improving dental health:

1. Oral health is closely affected not only by manpower arrangements, but also by consumer behaviour and beliefs.
2. Utilization of dental services in the areas studied does not reduce the incidence of dental disease.
3. The availability and accessibility of even the best system does not ensure good utilisation by the public.
4. The findings in adults indicate that even a well organized, widely available, school-based service does not necessarily lead to a satisfactory level of oral health in adult life.

The analysis of the data from the International Collaborative Study[2] has some important policy implications. The main one is that the preventive efforts of the public and the profession are both important but, as yet, inadequate. Some countries provide a school dental service for children and subsequently leave them to seek private dental treatment as adults. Other countries encourage children and adults to attend the same dentist throughout life. This encourages continuity of care.

There are few differences in the effectiveness of these alternative systems when judged by their ability to prevent tooth loss in middle-age. Whilst this is generally true, some individuals benefit from each system. This suggests that no single method of dental care is suited to all sections of a population. A number of methods should be available and each should have equal status and not be identified with a particular socio-economic group. The study points to the importance of involving consumers in discussions concerning the acceptability of dental care.

The study also highlights the relationship between a repair-oriented dental service, the rate of dental disease, the way adults pay for dental care and the socio-economic status of the community. In countries with health insurance and private payment systems, a small part of the population takes up a large part of dentist's time and the financial resources.

These findings are portentious: they suggest that, in the absence of broadly based preventive measures, an increasingly greater proportion of resources will be devoted to technical procedures on a smaller segment of the population. Important steps in reversing these trends will include prevention on a wide scale; a change in philosophy of restorative dentists and the organisation of dental services which are acceptable and accessible to all. These measures require an extensive programme of public health education to encourage a change of diet, fluoridation of water supplies or supplementary fluorides, and the improvement of oral hygiene. In addition, the public should be involved in the planning of dental services which should be an integral part of the general health service.

The second insight into the shortcomings of the present systems is provided by the significant decline in dental caries in children in most industrialized countries in the past 10 years.[22] The reasons for the decline are considered to be an increasing use of fluoridated toothpaste, a decrease in the consumption of added sugars, improved oral cleanliness and anti-biotics used for medical or veterinary pur-poses. So the major factors in the im-provement in dental health are related to changes in the behaviour of the popula-tion which are not health-directed, al-though they are health-related. The treat-ment model of dental care, with the em-phasis on attempted cure of existing dis-ease and individualistic remedies and pre-ventive approaches, has played a minor role in these changes. Moreover, the im-provements in dental health has caused some concern among dental associations because dentists are not finding enough treatment to carry out. Unless there is a major change in philosophy, treatment-oriented dentists will transfer their atten-tions from restorative dentistry to techni-cal solutions to periodontal disease. This will increase the cost of dental services and undermine the preventive behaviours of the public by encouraging dependency on the dentist. In addition, the repeated scaling and root planing of shallow pock-ets will increase the rate of loss of attach-ment.[10]

The mechanistic attitude to people that leads to a manipulative engineering ap-proach, which is prevalent in dental ser-vices, is particularly inappropriate in the prevention and treatment of periodontal diseases. A behavioural holistic model of health behaviour is needed. The inappro-priateness is accentuated by the concen-tration on items of treatment and on the predominant fee for service system of payment.

Dental Health Services in Europe

In most European countries, national sys-tems of dental health care comprise three components: private, public and tran-sitional. The latter is usually represented by dental health insurance.[9] In private den-tal practice, dentists treat each case in what they consider is the best interests of the patient. They are independent and are paid directly by the patient. *Kostlan*[9] considers that this concept of oral health service is often at variance with that of modern dental health service systems which are founded on the need to satisfy the aspirations of large population groups. Dental health insurance is a modification of private dental practice. The dentist works as a private practitioner, but is paid for items of treatment carried out by a combination of either total payment by a third party, or by contributions from pa-tients and third parties. In this system, by changing the financial benefits for patients and the fees per item of service for the dentist, the pattern of behaviour and treat-ment can be influenced.

The dominant system of payment in both these systems is the fee-for-item of ser-vice. Most of the tariffs of fees encourage intervention rather than prevention and gives preference to curative procedures. Such a system of payment is inimical to rational periodontal care. It encourages the continuation of the individualistic mechanistic approach.

Alternative systems of payment, such as salary or capitation, do not have such shortcomings. Payment by salary is com-mon in public dental health services.

Since the ideology of a free profession is deeply rooted in many dental associa-tions, it is unlikely that they will willingly accept a salaried service. Capitation is the most appropriate system of payment for the dentist and for the community. This system is based on a payment for the maintenance of dental fitness.[5] It has the following advantages:

1. It encourages the maintenance of a healthy mouth.
2. It offers a more realistic standard by which to measure and reward increased effort by the dental team.

3. It encourages preventive dentistry and the teaching of oral hygiene since in contrast to the fee-for-item, a healthy mouth will be more profitable than an unhealthy one.
4. It encourages closer cooperation between the private dentist and the public health service. The more health education is carried out by the public health service, the less need there will be for the dentist to do prolonged and frequently unsuccessful dental health education.
5. It discourages intervention and encourages continuity of care.
6. It is relatively easy to administer and will facilitate rational planning of dental services for the whole population.

A dental care system should encourage those working in it to apply known effective methods to improve and maintain oral health for the population. It should be personally and financially satisfying and encourage innovation and the integration of efforts with other health and educational services and with the community. The existing dental health services in Europe do not have most of these characteristics. Small changes in the regulations and fee systems to encourage the treatment of periodontal disease is unlikely to improve oral health. More fundamental changes in the system of payment and the philosophy of dental care are required.

References

1. *Blinkhorn A. S.*
   Toothbrushing as part of primary socialization. Ph. D. Thesis. University of Manchester 1976.

2. *Cohen, L. K.*
   International comparisons in the provison of oral health care. Brit. Dent. J. 1980, 149: 347–351.

3. Committee Report, Structure and Metabolism of the Normal Periodontium. In International Conference on Research in the Biology of Periodontal Disease. The College of Dentistry, University of Illinois, Chicago, 1977, p89.

4. *Cowell C. R. and Sheiham A.*
   Promoting Dental Health. King Edward's Hospital Fund for London, 1981, p39.

5. General Dental Services Committee. Methods of remuneration. Report of Committee under the Chairmanship of W. R. Tattersall. Brit. Dent. J., 1964, 117: 331–346.

6. *Glavind L., Zeuner E. and Attström R.*
   Oral hygiene instruction of adults by means of a self-instructional manual. J. Clin. Periodontol., 1981, 8: 165–176.

7. *Hamp S. E and Johannsson L. A.*
   Dental prophylaxis for youths in their late teens. J. Clin. Periodontol., 1982, 9: 22–34.

8. *Hodge H. C., Holloway P. J. and Bell C. R.*
   Factors associated with toothbrushing behaviour in adolescents. Brit. Dent. J., 1982, 152: 49–51.

9. *Kostlan J.*
   Oral Health Services in Europe. WHO Regional Publications, European Series No. 5. WHO Regional Office for Europe, Copenhagen, 1979.

10. *Lindhe J., Westfeldt E., Nyman S., Socransky S. S., Heijl L. and Bratthall G.*
    Healing following surgical/non-surgical treatment of periodontal disease. A clinical study. J. Clin. Periodontol., 1982, 9: 115–128.

11. *Löe H., Anerud A., Boysen H. and Smith M.*
    The natural history of periodontal disease in man. J. Periodontol., 1978, 49: 607–620.

12. *MacPhee T. and Muir K. F.*
    The Contained Lesion and the Progressive Lesion in Periodontitis. In Efficacy of Treatment Procedures in Periodontitis. (Shanley D. ed.) Quintessence Publ. Co., Chicago, 1980, pp 175–190.

13. *Pilot T.*
    Analysis of the overall effectiveness of treatment of periodontal disease. In Efficacy of treatment Procedures in Periodontitis. (Shanley D. ed.) Quintessence Publ. Co., Chicago, 1980, pp 213–231.

14. *Ramfjord S. P.*
    Clinical research in periodontics. Proc. Finn. Dent. Soc., 1980, 76: 195–200.

15. *Rayner J. F. and Cohen L. K.*
    School dental health education. In Social Sciences and Dentistry. (Richards N. D. and Cohen L. K. eds.) Federation Dentaire Internationale, London, 1971, pp 275–307.

16. *Selikowitz H. S., Sheiham A., Albert D. and Williams G. M.*
    Retrospective longitudinal study of the rate of

alveolar bone loss in humans using bite-wing radiographs. J. Clin. Periodontol., 1981, 8: 431–438.

17. *Sheiham A.*
Prevention and Control of Periodontal Disease. In International Conference on Research in the Biology of Periodontal Disease. College of Dentistry, University of Illinois. Chicago, 1977, pp 309–368.

18. *Sheiham A.*
Current concepts in Health Education. In Efficacy of Treatment Procedures in Periodontics. (Shanley, D. ed.) Quintessence Publ. Co., Chicago, 1980, pp 23–34.

19. *Sheiham A.*
Promoting periodontal health: effective education promotion programmes. Int. Dent. J., 1983, 33: 182–187.

20. *Söderholm G.*
Effect of a dental care program on dental health conditions. University of Lund, Malmö, Sweden, 1979.

21. *Suomi J. D., Greene J. C., Vermillion J. R., Doyle J., Chang J. C. and Leatherwood E. C.*
The effect of controlled oral hygiene procedures on the progression of periodontal disease in adults: results after third and final year. J. Periodontol., 1971, 42: 152–160.

22. *von der Fehr, F.*
Dental disease in Scandinavia. In Dental Health Care in Scandinavia. (Frandsen A. ed.) Quintessence Publ. Co., Chicago, 1982, pp 21–43.

23. *WHO.*
Epidemiology, Etiology, and Prevention of Periodontal Diseases. Technical Report Series, WHO, Geneva, 1978.

24. *WHO.*
Principles and Methods of Health Education. European Report Series No. 11. WHO, Copenhagen, 1979.

5. Experiences in Periodontal Care under the Insurance System in West Germany

Lavinia Flores-de-Jacoby and Robert Jacoby

Historical Survey of Periodontal Insurance in the Federal Republic of Germany

The treatment of patients suffering from periodontal disease was being discussed in Germany as long ago as 60 years. Östmann had developed in 1925[13,3] at the Institute of Weski in Berlin, a periodontal record form on which the clinical and x-ray findings, as well as those of study casts, were to be entered.

The first 'guidelines' for the periodontal treatment of those who were socially insured were adopted at the ARPA Congress in Nürnberg in 1927. These 'guidelines' were recognized by the 'Reichsverband' in 1933 and the first insurance contracts for the treatment of 'paradontose' were subsequently made between the National Association of German Dentists Ltd. ('Reichsverband' der Zahnärzte Deutschlands e.V.) and the Association of Business Men's Health Insurance Companies (Verband kaufmännischer Berufskrankenkassen).[3]

The political events in 1933, with their catastrophic consequences for Germany, also had far-reaching repercussions on the scientific work of German dentists as well as on their social-political status.[3] The statutes of the 'Reichsverband' and of scientific societies were changed and brought into line with the NAZI ideology. After the war, the managing board of the Federal Association of Dentists participating in a health insurance plan strove to change the then existing periodontal record form.[3]

The duties imposed by the contractual regulations of the social insurance, and the resulting difficulties for dentists and students at various universities in using different printed forms, gave the impulse to work out a new status which would re-establish a uniformity in documentation and instruction.[2]

At the annual meeting of the German ARPA in Bad Harzburg in 1964, Schulte[21] presented a simplified model with a sketch of the clinical findings.

The Present Contracts with the Health Insurance Companies

This new status (periodontal record form), with some modifications, served as the basis for the new periodontal contracts with the health insurance companies in 1969[5] (contract between the Federal Association of Dentists participating in a health insurance plan [panel dentists] Ltd and the Association of Employees' Health Insurance Company [VDAK] as well as with the Workers' Health Insurance Company [AEV] and the National Insurance Company [RVO].)

The companies and the professional groups

In the Federal Republic of Germany, the systems of health insurance are as follows[24]:

1. The private health insurance companies.
2. The health insurance funds (Ersatzkassen and Arbeiter-Ersatzkassen).
3. The national insurance companies (RVO).

On the first of October 1982, the number of the private health insurance companies was 41. Besides these private insurance companies, there are approximately 90 smaller private insurance groups and benevolent funds under federal and state supervision. For the most part, they offer only supplemental support.

Among the health insurance funds (Ersatzkassen VdAK/AEV), there are 15 different companies (of these 7 are health insurance funds for employees 'VdAK' and 8 worker insurance funds 'AEV').

The National Insurance Companies consist of:

– The Compulsory Health Insurance Groups (270 different groups, AOK = Allgemeine Ortskrankenkasse)
– The Staff health insurance funds (825 different funds, BKK = Betriebskrankenkasse)
– The Guilds health insurance funds (155 different funds, IKK = Innungskrankenkasse)
– The Farmers' health insurance funds (19 different funds, LKK = Landwirtschaftliche Krankenkasse)
– The Sailor's insurance fund (1 company, Seekrankenkasse)
  Federal miner's fund (1 company, Bundesknappschaft)

Which Dentists May Treat a Periodontally Diseased Patient?

Any licenced dentist can carry out periodontal therapy. When a dentist establishes his own practice, he applies to the insurance companies to be allowed to treat patients who are socially insured. Should the dentist no longer be able to treat socially insured patients, he must inform the insurance company of this. A renewal of application will not be approved.

Which Patients May Be Treated Periodontally?

All patients who show symptoms of periodontal disease may be treated in the Federal Republic of Germany. The patient may select the dentist of his choice. The only prerequisite is that the dentist chosen has entered into contract with the appropriate insurance companies.

Guidelines

General considerations

The guidelines agreed upon by the Federal Committee of Dentists and Federal Insurance Companies attempt to assure a sufficient, suitable and economical dental care according to the National Insurance Law.

According to these guidelines, socially insured dental care comprises those measures suitable to heal diseases of the teeth, mouth and jaw according to the standards of medical practice, to alleviate complaints due to these diseases and to prevent deteriorations.

Measures which serve only cosmetic purposes do not belong in the preview of socially insured dental care.

In the framework of socially insured dental care, the panel dentist determines the type and scope of the measures employed. In this regard, he is to see to it that the means placed at his disposal by the insurance companies are sensibly used.

The work of a panel dentist falls under the heading of socially insured dental care even if he carries it out at the request of another panel doctor.

The panel dentist should only use those methods of examination and treatment whose diagnostic or therapeutic value is sufficiently recognized. The trying-out of new methods at the expense of the insurer is impermissible.

Those dentists who participate in socially insured dental care schemes are, moreover, to see to it that their substitutes and assistants know and heed these guidelines.

Guidelines for the systematic ascertainment of medical and dental findings and treatment of periodontal disease[4]

A systematic surgical treatment of periodontal disease must be preceded by a preliminary treatment carried out in accordance with the latest scientific findings.

The aims of the systematic treatment are:

to prevent disease progression, to abate inflammation, and to forestall further destruction of the periodontal tissues. According to these guidelines, a systematic periodontal treatment is advisable in the cases of:

– Parodontitis marginalis superficialis (Periodontitis levis)
– Parodontitis marginalis profunda (Periodontitis gravis and Periodontitis complicata) and
– Gingival recession

The treatment of gingivitis is not mentioned in this contract because it is treated with measures used only in the framework of preliminary treatment. This contract applies only to surgical treatment of periodontal disease.

All other measures (preliminary treatment) which are used before the surgical appointment or between surgical appointments do not belong to this contract and are remunerated according to conservative methods of treatment (e.g. cleaning of teeth, plaque-staining with disclosing substances).

Several pretreatment sessions may be necessary. In the framework of the preliminary treatment the cause and further possible progress of the disease is explained to the patient. He is also instructed on the proper method of cleaning his teeth. The removal of supragingival calculus, of soft debris and the elimination of factors of local irritation (defective fillings, caries) are also included in the preliminary treatment.

The dentist will wait 2 to 3 weeks after completion of the preliminary treatment in order to determine whether a systematic surgical periodontal treatment is called for. Should the patient prove himself willing to actively cooperate in his own oral hygiene care, and a successful outcome of the treatment be therefore expected, the dentist may then begin to draw up the necessary documents on findings insofar as the inflammatory process has not subsided during or after preliminary treatment[4].

The documentation of the findings required is as follows:

– A complete set of periodontal x-rays using a right angle technique if possible (panorama-shots or orthopanthomograms are not sufficient for the x-ray diagnosis of periodontal disease).
– The casting of models of the upper and lower jaws by which all of the tooth areas and also the vestibular area are to be exactly represented.
– The filling in of a periodontal record.

71

....	....
(Family name and first name of the member)	(Contracting insurance company)
....	....
(Family name and first name of the patient, birth date)	(Member's insurance number)
....	....
(complete address)	(A member since)

....

(Contracting insurance company)

....

(Member's insurance number)

....

(A member since)

....

(Employer)

Pensioner: .... yes / no ....

I. General medical history:

Diabetes? .... ☐
Vasomotoric illness .... ☐
Stomach or intestinal
disorders .... ☐

Other present illnesses: ....

....

....

Diagnoses:

....

....

....

Place   Date   Seal and signature of
                              the dentist

II. Dental History

ANUG?

once? .... ☐
more than once? .... ☐
Gingival-bleeding? .... ☐
Tendency towards the formation
of plaque? .... ☐
Tooth migrations? .... ☐
Tooth loss through mobility? .... ☐
Previous orthodontic treatment? ....

III. Findings:

A. Parafunctions and effects:

Bruxism? .... ☐
Pressing? .... ☐
Pressing of the lips? .... ☐
Pressing of the tongue? .... ☐
Abrasions? .... ☐

Other? ....

B. Removable denture? .... ☐
      for ...... years

Crowns and fixed bridges? .... ☐
      for ...... years

C. Marginal periodontitis:
Inflammation

                    general? .... ☐
                    localized? .... ☐
Sulcus exudate? .... ☐
Subgingival calculus? .... ☐

Opinion of the consultant (in case requested):

Consultant: ....

Address: ....

Street: ....

1. I (do not) recommend the assumption of costs.

2. Reason(s) for non-recommendation (if necessary on a separate sheet).

....

....

Place   Date   Seal and signature of
                              the consultant

Entry for the contracting Insurance company

The costs of the recommended systematic periodontal treatment will (not) be assumed.

....

....

....

Place   Date   Seal of the contracting insurance company

Fig. 5.1   Front side of periodontal record form.

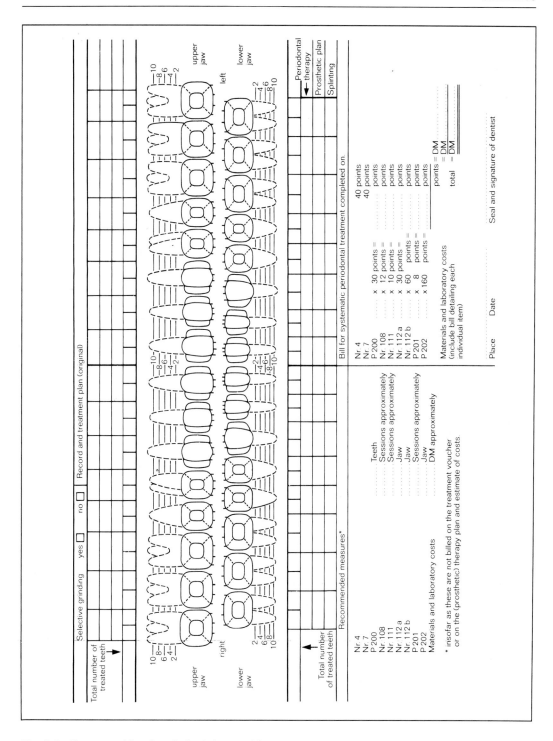

Fig. 5.2   Reverse side of periodontal record form.

The front side of this record (Fig. 5.1) contains, besides personal data and information about the patient's insurance, data concerning his past general medical history and his special dental history as well as the local findings. In addition, the diagnoses and the evaluation of an expert are entered.

On the reverse side of the periodontal record form (Fig. 5.2), information about missing teeth, teeth to be extracted, sulcus or pocket depths, gingival recession, caries and fillings, overhanging fillings, crowns and bridges, degree of tooth mobility, exposed bifurcations and trifurcations, nonvital teeth, root fillings, elongations, tiltings, migrations etc., are to be entered. The careful documentation of these findings is an indispensable prerequisite for the dentist's planning and carrying out of the periodontal treatment as well as for any consultant opinion.

The Double Expert Opinion System of the Insurance Companies

The dentist sends the completed periodontal form to the insurance company for approval. The insurance company may approve the treatment immediately; they may however also seek an expert opinion on the periodontal record. In this case, they will send the periodontal record back to the dentist and ask him to forward it together with the other findings (x-rays, models) to the consultant whom they have designated. The consultant may ask for further data as well as follow-up findings to be supplied by the dentist. The costs involved will be refunded to the dentist by the insurance company. The same holds true for the costs of the consultant.

The consultant then gives his opinion on the case. Should he recommend treatment, he will return the periodontal record to the insurance company. All other material he will send back to the dentist.

Should the consultant not recommend treatment, he will send the periodontal record back to the insurance company together with a written explanation of his reasons. The other materials will be returned to the dentist. The insurance company then returns the periodontal record to the dentist with the consultant's opinion and informs him that the insurance company will not pay for the costs of the treatment. Either the dentist or the insurance company may appeal the consultant's decision for review by a chief consultant.

The objection is to be recorded officially in the Federal Association of Panel Dentists within a period of 2 months after having received the consultant's decision.

These chief consultants are dentists experienced and active in the field of periodontology, or university professors of periodontology, and they are appointed as the highest authority by the Federal Union of Panel Dentists in agreement with the State Association of Insurance Companies. The costs of the chief consultant are generally paid by the insurance company. However, if the appeal is unsuccessful, then the panel dentist pays the costs of the chief consultant.

Coverage for a Systematic Periodontal Treatment

Together with the filling in of the periodontal record, an estimate of materials and services to be remunerated is made.

The actual settlement is, however, made only after therapy has been completed. The periodontal record also serves as the bill or statement of account.

Services rendered in a systematic surgical periodontal treatment:

Nr. 4   Fact-finding and the working out of a therapy and cost plan.

Nr. 7   Study casts of the upper and lower jaws.

P 200   Surgical treatment per tooth.
This treatment includes all measures of this type (e.g. subgingival curettage with root planing, gingivectomy, gingivoplasty, flap operations including suture and/or surgical dressing).
The anaesthesia is to be billed extra.

Nr. 108 Grindings per session (a maximum of 4 sessions).

Nr. 111 Follow-up treatment per session (change of dressing, removal of suture, cleaning the wound etc.).
(Maximum of 10 sessions).

Nr. 112a Splinting by means of ligature dressing, for each jaw.

Nr. 112b Temporary splinting per jaw (e.g. composites).

Nr. 201 Oral irrigation. This service had its historical origin in the oral washing ('oral shower') of *Weissenfluh.*
The instrument which succeeded this one was the *Paradento-Spray* of Dürr Dental.
According to established scientific findings, the effect of both instruments in periodontal therapy is zero.[20]

P 202   Miniplast-splints per jaw (thermoforming system).

Material and laboratory costs are presently fixed at about 15.00 DM. The financial settlement of such treatment is remunerated according to a fee system for every individual service. The value of the individual service is calculated according to an established point system. Each point has a present value of DM 1.16 to DM 1.25 depending on the insurance company. The estimate for pocket therapy is made according to the number of treated teeth. The teeth suffering from periodontal disease listed separately for the upper and lower jaws are to be added up and the sum entered at the bottom left. For example, a patient with 28 periodontally diseased teeth is examined and treated. In four sessions, occlusal interferences and serious premature contacts are removed by grinding the teeth. For the follow-up treatment the dentist needs six sessions. There is no splinting done.
We would then have:

Examination to determine the findings (Nr. 4)	40 Points
Castings of the upper and lower jaws (Nr. 7)	40 Points
28 periodontally diseased treated teeth (P 200) (30 Points per tooth)	840 Points
Grinding (4 sessions) (Nr. 108) (12 Points per session)	48 Points
Follow-up treatment (6 sessions) (Nr. 111) (10 Points per session)	60 Points
Total	1028 Points

The approximate point value is DM 1.16 (RVO 01. 07. 82).
The periodontal treatment for this patient would therefore cost the insurance company DM 1.192.48.

Brief Comments on Epidemiology

Epidemiological investigations in Düsseldorf, Hamburg, Hannover, Kiel and Saarbrücken between 1970 and 1975 established that over 85% of the German population between the ages of 7 and 87 suffer from some form of periodontal disease.[15, 16, 17, 18, 19] A study of the periodontal condition, as well as of the composition of the subgingival microflora of Marburg children aged 12 to 14 years, showed that neither those who wore orthodontic appliances nor the nonwearers (the control group) exhibited healthy clinical and microbiological periodontal conditions.[6, 7, 10, 12]

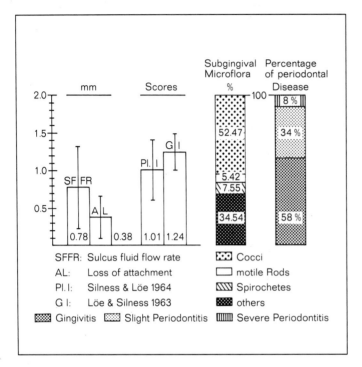

Figure 5.3

Further clinical and microbiological investigations of a select group of 100 preclinical dental students aged 18 to 29 years who come from various states in the Federal Republic, showed that no student could be regarded as periodontally healthy.[8, 9] (Fig. 5.3)

According to these figures, one must assume that almost every German adult is suffering from periodontal disease.

Number of periodontal treatments carried out in the Federal Republic of Germany

Table 5.1 shows the number of periodontal treatments carried out in the Federal Republic of Germany.[22, 23, 24, 25]

One of the reasons for this low treatment level can be found in the dental curricula. Even today the field of periodontology is taught by either conservative or surgical departments, the exceptions being at the Universities of Münster and Marburg. (However, lecture courses in periodontology have recently been started in six additional West German universities.)

In comparison with other European countries and the USA, periodontal instruction is under-represented in the curricula of German universities.[11] Except for the removal of calculus and the filling out of the periodontal record, there is in many places no further periodontal training done. A good number of young German dentists leave university without receiving any instruction in this important field, not to mention ever having been examined in it. Should the already licensed dentist later want to take a postgraduate course in periodontology, he will be facing a similar situation. Except for the possibility of taking a postgraduate course in one of the aforementioned universities, he can only acquire some knowledge and practical ex-

Table 5.1 Periodontal Treatments in the Federal Republic of Germany.

Year	Number of Dentists	Periodontally treated patients	Number of periodontally treated patients per dentist %
1970	31708	6000	0.18
1974	33022	30000	0.98
1975	33472	82835	2.47
1980	34339	159557	4.64
1981	34739	179812	5.14

perience if he becomes an assistant to a dentist who himself does periodontal therapy. Unfortunately, there are still too few such centres of education. If young graduates have insufficient qualifications for the practical application of periodontal methods, how much worse must the situation be among the older colleagues?

Those who do not acquire the necessary knowledge during their course of training – and this can be done only at the cost of a considerable effort – must remain passive bystanders.

At this point, some critical remarks must be made about further education for dentists. Although every dentist is obliged to continue his education according to the statutes of the dental society, only a small proportion of colleagues manage to fulfil this obligation sufficiently. As long as we are unable to reach large sections of practising dentists with postgraduate dental courses, no general improvement of the situation may be expected. In addition, not all of the courses in continued education which are offered are indeed particularly worthwhile.

For example, lecture courses given to colleagues with no or limited practical experience in periodontology are of questionable value.

This insufficient training and lack of even the very basics of periodontal knowledge is especially astonishing among col-leagues who have been appointed as 'experts' by the state confederations of panel dentists for the purpose of giving expert opinions on periodontal cases submitted to the insurance companies for approval by practising dentists.

A further reason for this small number of periodontal treatments is the patient himself with his apathy and carelessness. On the one hand, he lacks the necessary motivation and information and on the other he fails to recognize the necessity of treatment when he is not in obvious pain. In addition to this, the patient is seldom able to fulfill the prerequisites for a successful periodontal treatment, that is the maintenance of good oral hygiene.

The lack of dental hygienists in the Federal Republic of Germany is also of enormous importance. These hygienists could help in pretreatment and in the check-ups after periodontal treatment by, for example, removing supra- and subgingival soft and hard deposits.

But in the Federal Republic of Germany there are no centres of education for 'dental hygienists'. Efforts, however, have been made to encounter this problem by opening schools for 'dental assistants'. In this course of instruction, which lasts 6 months, the dental nurse acquires the theoretical knowledge and practical experience which will be advantageous in a periodontal practice.

This training is of course not to be compared with the 2 year training of an American or Swiss dental hygienist.

Advantages of This System

For the patients

One appreciable advantage (and we believe the greatest one of this system) is without a doubt that the socially insured patient who is periodontally diseased can receive 'adequate' systematic treatment and that the costs will be paid for by the insurance company. The same holds true for the postoperative check-ups recommended by the guidelines of these contracts where it was set down that because of the tendency of periodontally treated patients to have gingival inflammation, regular check-ups are in principle necessary after surgical treatment. These postoperative check-ups are also supposed to serve as a supervision of the patient's maintenance of oral hygiene and afford the opportunity of repeating local measures (the removal of hard and soft deposits), if necessary surgical measures on the individual periodontally diseased sites. It is recommended that the first postoperative check-up be carried out at the very latest 3 months after completion of the surgical treatment and that the interval between check-ups as a rule be no longer then 6 months.

Advantages for the dentist carrying out treatment

For the dentist who carries out treatment there are also considerable advantages with this system. Through these contracts the dentist has aquired freedom in the application of periodontal surgical measures. The contracts have intentionally departed from the practice of laying down special methods of treatment for certain cases.

This is now left to the responsibility, experience and ability of the individual dentist. What is important is that the aim of treatment is achieved and that the generally accepted principles of therapy (p. 70) are observed.

Advantages for the community

After the periodontal contracts were made and information was made available to the patients in the form of leaflets provided by the insurance companies, the interest of patients in undergoing periodontal treatment as well as the willingness of colleagues to undertake periodontal treatment increased. This was a result of both successful publicity and efforts on the part of colleagues to further their education in this area.

Postgraduate education courses in periodontology have, especially in the last 5 years, been increasingly offered by the Federal and State Dental Associations, the periodontal departments of universities, centres for further education, the Free Association of German Dentists and by the other scientific societies such as 'The New Group' and the German Society of Periodontology.

By helpfully advising the practising dentist, the consultants appointed by the state dental insurance companies have also contributed to the increase in periodontally treated patients and to the increase in dentists now actively carrying out periodontal treatment.

Disadvantages of This System

Concerning the success of the treatment on the part of the patient

This system unfortunately has disadvantages.

The generosity of the insurance companies in paying for all the charges for periodontal surgical treatment leads more often than not to a lack of cooperation on the part of the patient. The patient usually assumes that he does not need to clean his teeth thoroughly and regularly as the dentist will do this for him as often as it is really necessary.

He also assumes, falsely, that the dentist is in some way obliged to do so. The results of such an attitude are inevitably the failure of the periodontal treatment. As discussed earlier, such a lack of cooperation is a sufficient reason for refusing periodontal treatment. Another disadvantage is the unwillingness on the part of the patient to invest in the materials necessary to the maintenance of his own dental health. Toothbrushes, dentifrice, dental floss and disclosing wafers are not paid for by the insurance companies and so the patient does not buy them regularly.

Approximately 50% of the population do not brush their teeth or even possess a toothbrush.

Disadvantages with regard to the dentist

The dentist's lack of periodontal knowledge and of practical experience in this field results in teeth being extracted which could have been saved through periodontal treatment. There are still innumerable dentists in the Federal Republic of Germany whose only answer to the periodontally diseased patient seeking help is: 'There is nothing one can do about periodontal disease. Sooner or later your teeth are going to fall out anyway'.

Should a dentist proceed to treat a patient periodontally, one of the main reasons for its failure is the absence of any plaque-control programme on his part. Here it is the dentist who reckons with the generosity of the insurance companies. No check-up is made to find out whether the alleged periodontal treatment was carried out systematically and correctly. Often a hasty

and imperfect removal of supragingival deposits is billed as a periodontal treatment.

Disadvantages with respect to the insurance companies and the contracts

A lack of acceptance of the latest scientific findings led to the incorrect assertion of the traditional aetiological triad of Weski,[1] as the origin and development of periodontal disease. As a result, many dentists who are still unfortunately unaware of the scientific findings in the field of periodontology over the past 10 years try to hold up the process of periodontal disease (gingival inflammation, deep pockets, gingival recession) or even to prevent it from occurring by 'selectively' grinding down the teeth instead of getting rid of the inflammation as urgently as possible by means of local periodontal treatment. There is one area where the insurance companies will have to catch up on: until now, they have not deemed it necessary to remunerate either preventive measures or the time-consuming explanations and sessions of the dentist with regard to oral hygiene and prophylactic measures.

It was a great mistake on the part of the insurance companies to introduce the remuneration of all prosthetic measures before having granted payment for prophylactic measures.

The attempt on the part of the insurance companies to check-up on dental treatment by means of the 'investigatory board' discriminates precisely against those colleagues in underdeveloped areas who endeavour to employ mainly prophylactic, endodontic and periodontal measures. In these areas, the meaning of the words, prophylaxis, endodontics and periodontology are practically unknown.

It might happen that a dentist submitting his bill to the insurance company for work done for one year's quarter will include 20 root canals, 4 x-ray sets and 2 periodontal treatments which, in this area, means that these methods of treatment are 200% above the average. These investigatory boards are not accustomed to dentists performing root canals, periodontal treatment or making a complete systematic set of x-rays. The only things they are used to are extractions and dentures.

Recommendations for Improvement

For the dentists

As the majority of dentists have neither been taught the basics of oral structural biology, or of periodontal pathology, nor have had any practical training in these areas during their studies and professional training at university, the two possible ways of rectifying this situation would be firstly to offer further education courses over a period of several weeks, as is done in the USA, or in one or two week seminars as in Switzerland. Intensive weekend seminars are also very practicable. The other possibility would be a 1 or 2 year postgraduate course in periodontics at a university which has a department of periodontology. This course would either be financed by means of a fellowship or out of one's own resources, as in the USA.

The number and the quality of further education courses in periodontology, with practical demonstrations by periodontologists or dentists active in this field, must be intensified before any improvement in the present catastrophic situation may be expected.

For future dentists

Periodontology must finally be taught at all West German universities to an extent proportional to its importance. The curricula of the universities of Marburg and Münster, the only universities having independent departments of periodontology, have shown that it is easily possible to give at least 260 hours of instruction in periodontology within the framework of a complete course of studies lasting 10 semesters and using only those facilities and personnel presently available. For example, in Marburg, 7 hours are taught by Professor *Lehmann* during the pre-clinical studies. The rest of the hours must be taken during the five clinical semesters. This development was only possible owing to the support and assistance given to me by the managing director, the head of the prosthetic dentistry department and the head of the preventive dentistry section. A further recommendation would be the intensifying of periodontal research in the Federal Republic of Germany.

Introduction of preventive measures

An essential preliminary to any periodontal treatment is giving the patient absolutely necessary information and instructing him in the ways in which he must cooperate if the treatment is to have any hope of success. This takes up a great deal of time. It is not right to expect that the dentist will perform this service gratis.

In order to make such instruction in prophylactics more generally available to patients, it will have to be reimbursed. Naturally, it is only sensible to give such instruction to those patients who prove themselves really interested. In order to meet this requirement, the patient could, for example, request a voucher from the insurance company as is done in the case of medical check-ups. This would then entitle him to a half-an-hour of instruction in oral prophylactics.

In any case, this is one way in which a necessary and also effective prophylaxis of periodontal disease may be achieved.

It may be hoped that the goal will eventually be attained through federal and state health and education policies. The additional expenses accruing from the introduction of preventive measures, information and instruction will in the long run prove to be far more economical. It is also simpler and not painful for the patient.

Introduction into the contracts of provision for postoperative periodontal check-ups

In these check-ups the measurement of gingival inflammation, plaque and the documentation of these control findings (sulcus depths, tooth mobility) are indispensable. The repeated motivation of the patient is also most essential for the success of the already completed periodontal treatment. In most cases, a scaling is necessary. These measures take about two hours per session to complete.

Improvement in the periodontal record form

Changes which have occurred as a result of the latest research findings and of documented clinical experience must finally be taken into consideration. In particular, this means a much more precise periodontal examination and specification of the findings and finally the recognition of plaque as being the principle aetiological factor in the origin and development of periodontal disease. It means the use in diagnostics of parameters, which give detailed information about the periodontal condition of the patient (SFFR, attachment loss, composition of the subgingival microflora). These changes also require further education on the part of the consultants appointed by the state dental association; higher standards should be used for the selection of these experts and not only for the periodontological experts but especially for the prosthesis plans for periodontally treated cases.

Creation of training centres for dental assistants

The creation of centres for the education and training of dental assistants, who during the preliminary treatment and the recall appointments check and correct the patient's oral hygiene, is necessary. The further training of these assistants to perform subgingival scaling would be enormously helpful.

Provision for subgingival scaling and root planing

The guidelines should be changed to include a provision for subgingival scaling and root planing. As there are to date no provisions for these activities in the guidelines, they are not performed.

Conclusion

In conclusion, one might state that the present contracts in spite of the above mentioned advantages and disadvantages, neither promote nor secure the periodontal health of the population. The reasons for this are various: lack of periodontal instruction and training during the university education of German dentists and, on the other hand, the behaviour patterns of the population with regard to nutrition habits and oral hygiene. The fundamental question is whether it would not be better to invest the spent billions in prophylaxis instead of repairing damages.

Even if the necessary reform of dental studies were carried out and a drastic change in the oral hygiene and nutrition habits of the population took place, it would take years for tangible results to be seen.

References

1. *Bertzbach K.*
Die wissenschaftlichen Grundlagen der heutigen Pa-Behandlung und ihr Niederschlag in den Richtlinien für die systematische Pa-Behandlung. Dtsch. zahnärztl. Z., 1970, 25: 470–480.

2. *Bertzbach K.*
Der Parodontalstatus. In Deutscher Zahnärzte Kalender. Carl Hanser Verlag, München 1971, pp. 66–72.

3. *Bertzbach K.*
Geschichte der ARPA–DGP (1924–1974). Deutsche Gesellschaft für Parodontologie (DGP) e.V., VR 4685 Köln. Kösel, Kempten, 1982. pp. 37, 59, 201.

4. Bundesmantelvertrag für Zahnärzte (adenum F/ II/1). Kassenzahnärztliche Bundesvereinigung. Köln 1st. Jan., 1981.

5. Der neue PA-Vertrag mit den Ersatzkassen. Zahnärztliche Mitteilungen, 1969, pp. 870–884.

6. *Flores-de-Jacoby L., Hartmann F.* and *Jahn I.*
Untersuchung über den parodontalen Zustand jugendlicher Träger herausnehmbarer kieferorthopädischer Geräte (Klinische Studie). Dtsch. zahnärztl. Z., 1982, 37: 580–584.

7. *Flores-de-Jacoby L.* and *Müller H.-P.*
Zusammensetzung der subgingivalen Mundflora bei Trägern herausnehmbarer kieferorthopädischer Geräte und Nichtträgern. Dtsch. zahnärztl. Z., 1982, 37: (in Press).

8. *Flores-de-Jacoby L.* and *Rex M.*
The periodontal condition of the pre-clinic dental students in Marburg. (A clinical study) (to be published).

9. *Flores-de-Jacoby L.* and *Günther M.*
The composition of the subgingival microflora of the pre-clinic dental students in Marburg. 1982 (to be published).

10. *Hartmann F., Jeromin R.* and *Flores-de-Jacoby L.*
Untersuchung über den parodontalen Zustand jugendlicher Träger festsitzender kieferorthopädischer Geräte (Klinische Studie). Dtsch. zahnärztl. Z., 1982, 37: 585–589.

11. *Lange D. E.*
Zur Situation der Parodontologie in der Bundesrepublik Deutschland. Zahnärzt. Mitt., 1974, pp. 578–579.

12. *Müller H.-P.* and *Flores-de-Jacoby L.*
Zusammensetzung der subgingivalen Mundflora bei Trägern festsitzender kieferorthopädischer Geräte. Dtsch. zahnärztl. Z., 1982, 37: 855–860.

13. *Östman B.*
Das Parodontose Modell. Zahnärztliche Rundschau, 1925, Heft Nr. 11 pp. 1–4.

14. Paragraph 14 des Bundesmantelvertrages für Zahnärzte. Leitfaden für Gutachter (adenum 1. 3[2]). Stand 1. 10. 1981. Kassenzahnärztliche Vereinigung Westfalen-Lippe, 1982.

15. Parodontose Untersuchung in Saarbrücken. Zahnärztl. Mitt., 1970, pp. 717.

16. Parodontose Untersuchung. 87 Prozent Zahnbetterkrankungen in Hamburg. Zahnärztl. Mitt., 1973, pp. 189.

17. Parodontose Untersuchung in Düsseldorf. Zahnärztl. Mitt., 1973, pp. 579.

18. Parodontose Untersuchung in Kiel. Zahnärztl. Mitt., 1974, pp. 107.

19. Parodontose Untersuchung in Hannover. Zahnärztl. Mitt., 1974, pp. 867.

20. *Renggli H. H.*
Einfluß des Paradento-Sprays (R) auf Schmelz und Plaque. Schweiz. Monatsschr. Zahnheilkd., 1969, 79: 852–862.

21. *Schulte W.*
Zur Frage der Befundaufzeichnung bei marginalen Erkrankungen. Zahnärztl. Mitt., 1964, pp. 1102–1107.

22. Statistik der Zahnärzte. Stand 31. 3. 1971 Deutscher Zahnärzte Kalender. Carl Hanser Verlag, München, 1972, pp. 20.

23. Statistik der Zahnärzte. Stand 30. 09. 1974 Deutscher Zahnärzte Kalender. Carl Hanser Verlag, München 1975, pp. 299.

24. Statistik der Zahnärzte und der Krankenkassen. Personal Information from the Federal Committee of Dental Insurance (KZBV, Mrs. Gürtler), Köln, 8th October, 1982.

25. *Trefz H-J.*
Die Parodontal-Behandlung integriert in die tägliche Praxis. Zahnärztl. Mitt., 1976, pp. 221–224.

6. Attitudes and Behaviour with Respect to Oral Hygiene and Periodontal Treatment Needs in Selected Groups in West Germany

Dieter E. Lange

Introduction

In his search for epidemiological data regarding periodontal diseases in West Germany, Curilovic[11] concluded that the number of studies were limited.[3, 18, 24, 25,26, 53, 54, 57] However, there was a considerable amount of information concerning the explosive increase of costs, insurance problems and the efficiency of the national insurance fund (Krankenkasse). The problem of prevention and treatment of periodontal diseases was scarcely dealt with. This becomes obvious if one analyses the expenses for various dental services in 1980. According to a survey conducted by the 'Social Insurance System' the total costs of dental services amounted to 12.180.59 million DM. The financial contribution for periodontal diseases was 1.2%, or 148 million DM. At the same time the expenses for gold used in dentistry alone were about 1.200 million DM or eight times the cost of periodontal treatment measures. If the amounts tallied for the various insurance funds are expressed in absolute numbers, the yearly cost for periodontal treatment comes to 1 US Dollar per person (Table 6.1).

The German 'Social Insurance System' has failed to establish preventive aspects in dentistry. It has been and still is the general policy of the insurance system to give the insured members the opportunity to receive extensive restorative treatment of the highest quality, involving mainly crown and bridgework. On the average, 8 US Dollars worth of gold was spent for every insured patient in 1980. As a result of the restorative aspect of German dentistry – the overtreatment, on the one hand, and the absence of organized prophylaxis programmes on the other – the expectation for caries reduction and higher percentages of gingivitis-free and periodontitis-free dentitions is rather poor.

Due to the special situation in dentistry there is a tremendous lack of statistical data concerning dental awareness, attitudes and behaviour as regards oral hygiene and the actual need for periodontal treatment. Little research has so far been carried out in West Germany concerning the periodontal health of the general population. A broad epidemiological study has been in progress since 1978.[9, 24, 25, 26, 40, 56, 57, 60, 61] Some of our findings are presented here.

The prevalence and severity of periodontal disease increase with age. This relationship suggests that this disease is a cumulative process which begins in childhood and adolescence and would be most appropriately prevented at an early age.[35] The frequency and the severity of periodontal disease correlates with age,[29, 31, 32, 33] poor oral hygiene[2, 30, 41, 49] and the socio-economic level of the population.[39]

Table 6.1 Expenditure for dental services, compiled by the Social Insurance System.

Total costs of dental services	1980 in Mill. DM	
	12 180,59	Percent of total
Operative Dentistry and Oral Surgical Treatment	3 854,93	31,6 %
Prosthodontics	6 965,96	57,2 %
Orthodontics	1 203,13	9,9 %
Periodontal Treatment	148,43	1,2 %
Fractures of the jaws	8,14	0,1 %

Epidemiological Data on Attitudes and Behaviour with Respect to Oral Hygiene and Periodontal Treatment Needs

In order to obtain exact epidemiological data on the incidence and the degree of severity of marginal periodontal diseases in West Germany, various populations and age groups were examined. The final evaluation was done on 15-year-old pupils, 20-year-old army recruits, and 35-year-old residents of a university city in West Germany.

The Bottrop Study (children aged 14–15 years)

One hundred and fifty-six pupils were examined, of whom half were boys and half girls. The average age of the subjects was 14.6-years-old. Altogether 65.000 measurements were taken as a basis for this examination.[60, 61]

Results

About 35% exhibited scores 1 to 4 using Russell's Periodontal Index. Fifteen per cent presented scores 1 to 2.5 for the Sulcus-Bleeding-Index. About 45% of the subjects had pocket depths greater than 2 mm. The Plaque-Index, as described by *Quigley* and *Hein*,[41] was between 1 and 4 in approximately 75% of the cases (Table 6.2).

The population was divided into three socio-economic groups, based on family income, and a comparison was made between these and the clinical measurements. The classification of the socioeconomic groups in this study was made according to monthly family income: Group 1: DM 1.599 (low income) = SES 1; Group 3: DM 1.600 to DM 2.399 (medium income) = SES 3; Group 5: more than DM 2.400 (high income) = SES 5.

Caries, gingivitis and periodontal diseases were found to the same extent among both boys and girls. They were relatively widespread among high school students as well as secondary school pupils and at all socio-economic levels. The caries incidence amounted to a total of 90.4%. There was a negligible difference between the values found among secondary school groups (90.1%) as compared to high school students (91.1%). In considering the average number of carious teeth, however, it was found that the greater percentage of carious lesions was in the lower socio-economic class (SES 1). This group had an average of 5.43 carious le-

Table 6.2 Results of the Bottrop Study. DMFT-index, SBI, pocket depths, plaque-index and PI were determined. The subjects were classified according to the type of school attended and by socio-economic status.

	Frequency: percent subjects				
	Secondary School	High School	Socioeconomic Status		
			1	3	5
Caries	91,1	90,1	5,43 DMFT	–	3,98 DMFT
SB-Index 0,1–0,5	48,5	87,3	55,8	82,3	76,4
SB-Index 1,1–2,5	25,0	0,9	24,4	–	0
Quigley-Hein-Index (0,5)	6,6	39,0	9,0	44,4	42,2
Pocket depth > 2 mm	64,6	34,3	55,1	–	36,0
Periodontal Index (Russel) no pathological changes (< 2,0)	2,2	17,1	7,1	–	20,0
Periodontal Index (Russel) Pathological changes (> 2,0)	31,7	1,8	24,0	16,5	0

sions compared to 3.98 in the SES-class 5. The same results were found when secondary school pupils and high school students were compared.

Similar differences with regard to the social levels can be determined when the Sulcus-Bleeding-Index is used. SB-Index scores from 0.1 to 0.5 first were considered. This indicated a slight bleeding tendency. The majority of such pupils were in SES-Group 5 (75.4%) and SES-group 3 (82.3%). Only 55.8% were to be found in the low socio-economic group SES 1. In evaluating secondary school pupils and high school students 48.5% of the former were found to have low SBI-scores as compared to 87.3% of the high school students.

If, however, the higher SBI-scores of 1.1 to 2.5 indicating very high bleeding tendency were considered, then the following results were determined. In the higher SES Group 5, no SBI-score greater than 1 was found, whereas in the lower SES-Group 1, 24.4% had such scores. Among high school students only 0.9% showed a very high bleeding tendency, among 25% of secondary school children this was the case.

A thoroughly plaque-free dentition was not found in any of the pupils, but there were definite differences in terms of the degree of cleanliness within the social classes and the types of schools. While 42.2% of SES Group 5 and 44.4% of Group 3 had plaque scores of 0.5 or less, only 9% of Group 1 had such scores. In contrast only 6.6% of the secondary schoolers, as compared to 39% of the high school students, had low plaque scores of 0.5.

In evaluating the changes in the periodontal tissues and determining the Periodontal Index (PI), it was observed that a total of 87.2% of the pupils exhibited periodontal lesions. When pocket depths were measured it was found that in SES Group 5 only 36% of the pupils had pockets deeper than 2 mm; in the lower socio-economic group (SES 1) this was the case in 55.1%. 34.3% of the high school students had 1 or more pockets deeper than 2 mm, among the secondary school children the percentage was twice as high (64.6%).

The evaluation of the Periodontal Index (PI) reveals that no pathological changes are seen in 20% of the individuals with a higher socio-economic status (SES 5). Here again the situation is less favourable in SES Group 1: only 7.1% showed no pathological changes. The comparison of school types revealed that 17.1% of high school students are free of such pathology, whereas only 2.2% of secondary school children had a PI below 2.0.

PI-Index values greater than 2, indicating considerable pathological changes, were found in 24% of persons in SES Group 1, 6.5% in SES Group 3, and none were found in SES Group 5. In analysing the data among pupils, it was shown that only 1.8% of those in high school had diseased conditions, while 31.7% of secondary school pupils had considerable pathological changes.

The income factor can therefore be considered the most important component of socio-economic status (SES). The concept has been confirmed in other studies,[43, 44, 45, 46, 47] that diseases of the teeth and oral cavity, particularly dental caries and periodontal disease, are dependent on socio-economic status.[17, 38, 39] Our study demonstrated similar findings in West Germany. The results of the Periodontal-Index confirm that diseases of the periodontal tissues occur more frequently in highly industrialized countries than in less industrialized areas. The total PI determined in this study was 87.2%, which is far greater than the values of studies made in Singapore and India.[17, 38] This is re-lated to two factors which can be seen as consequences of modern civilization; eating habits and extremely inadequate oral hygiene practices which are not being made to compensate for the increased consumption of sugar. The high caries incidence of 90.4% found in this study corresponds to the findings of other authors. The direct relationship between the development of gingivitis and periodontal disease and oral hygiene habits is undisputed. Although none of the pupils' dentition was totally free of plaque, there were definite differences in the degree of cleanliness seen within the social classes and school types.

The Dortmund Study (children aged 14 to 16 years)

For the purpose of an international multi-centre study,[16, 29] in which 12 countries participated and which was supported by the World Health Organization WHO, a total of 647 children, 342 girls and 305 boys, between the ages of 14 and 16 years, from schools in the Dortmund area, were examined.[25, 40] Bitewing x-rays in the first molar area were taken and plaque and inflammation indices were established. In addition, pocket depths were measured on the Ramfjord-teeth. The DMF-index was also determined. The x-rays were evaluated using an x-ray viewscreen. If the measure of the distance between the cementoenamel junction and the crest of the alveolar bone was greater than 2 mm, the condition was defined as bone loss.

Results

The results of the clinical evaluation showed that the molar groups had a plaque-index (*Silness* and *Löe*) of 1.3, while in the anterior tooth area a 0.83 value occurred (Fig. 6.1).

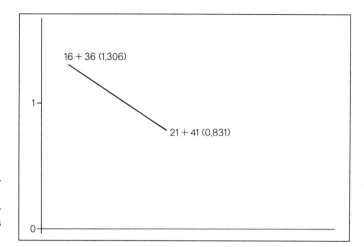

Fig. 6.1 Evaluation of Plaque-Indices. The index for teeth 21 and 41 was 0.831, for the molars 16 and 36 the index was 1.306.

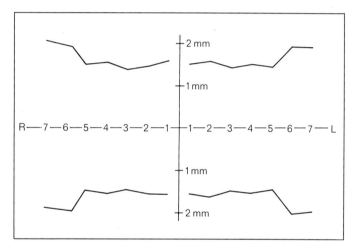

Fig. 6.2 Pocket depths. In the area of the molars the average pocket depths were about 0.5 mm deeper than around the premolars and anterior teeth.

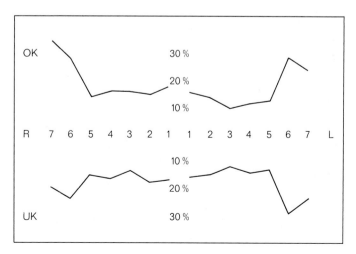

Fig. 6.3 Evaluation of the SBI (%).

Table 6.3 Multicentre Study. Results from West Germany: 10.4% of the children investigated showed bone loss.

Bone loss	male (%)	female (%)	total (%)
Horizontal	14 (5,4)	19 (6,1)	33 (5,8)
Vertical	6 (2,3)	20 (6,5)	26 (4,6)
Total	20 (7,7)	39 (12,6)	59 (10,4)

The average pocket depths were about 0.5 mm deeper in the molar area than around the premolars and anterior teeth. Sulcus depths of 2 mm were observed in 51.9% of the investigated 647 children while 7.35% of them had 3 mm deep pockets (Fig. 6.2). The molars exhibited a 10% greater Sulcus-Bleeding-Index than the anterior teeth and premolars (Fig. 6.3). The results of the x-ray evaluations showed that horizontal and vertical bone destruction had occurred in 10.4% of the cases (Table 6.3).

The findings of the Dortmund study correspond with those of the multicentre study.[16, 29] A prevalence of 10% or more subjects with bone destruction (Table 6.4) at the age of 15 years is therefore not uncommon.

Epidemiological Investigation of Army Recruits (Aged 20 Years)

The following data was collected for 143 20-year-old recruits of the German Army. This study was part of a multicentre study designed to evaluate oral hygiene condition and periodontal treatment needs of recruits.[6, 7, 8, 10, 15, 21, 26, 28, 34, 48, 56, 57]

Assessment of the data included:

1. Determination of the Periodontal Disease Index.
2. Determination of the extent of gingival inflammation (SBI)
3. Determination of the amount of plaque present (according to the Quigley-Hein Plaque-Index).
4. Amount of calculus present.
5. Measurement of the periodontal pocket depths.

Table 6.4 Percentage of 15-year-old children from 12 different geographic locations with bone loss on bite-wing radiographs (from Gjermo[16]).

INTERNATIONAL BITE-WING INVESTIGATION (1979 – 1980)

Individuals with bone loss (in %)

Country	N	Horizontal			Vertical			Total		
		M	F	T	M	F	T	M	F	T
DK	483	4,8	4,3	4,6	0,8	1,7	1,2	5,6	6,0	5,8
GDR	281	18,1	9,7	13,2	0,9	2,4	1,8	19,0	12,1	14,9
SF	383	9,8	3,4	6,8	0,0	0,0	0,0	9,8	3,4	6,8
THAI	393	20,8	12,8	16,0	2,0	1,3	1,6	22,8	14,1	17,6
BRA₁	164	1,9	9,0	6,7	3,8	1,8	2,4	5,7	10,8	9,1
N	2077	15,2	9,4	12,2	0,5	0,7	0,6	15,7	10,1	12,8
BRA₂	177	10,3	5,9	7,3	0,0	1,7	1,1	10,3	7,6	8,4
FRG	570	5,4	6,1	5,8	2,3	6,5	4,6	7,7	12,6	10,4
JAP	171	15,5	8,2	12,9	0,0	1,6	0,6	15,5	9,8	13,5
CH	182	0,0	0,0	0,0	2,2	1,1	1,6	2,2	1,1	1,6
BRA₃	38	35,7	8,3	18,4	0,0	8,3	5,3	35,7	16,6	23,7
TK	182	10,0	9,8	9,9	0,0	3,3	1,6	10,0	13,1	11,5

(DK – Denmark, GDR – German Democratic Republic, SF – Finland, THAI – Thailand, BRA – Brazil, N – Norway, FRG – Federal Republic of Germany, JAP – Japan, CH – Switzerland, TK – Turkey.)

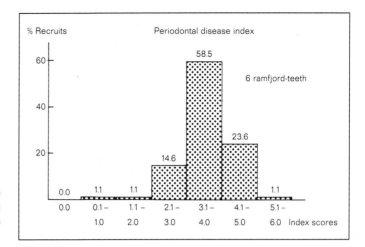

Fig. 6.4 Distribution of the subjects examined according to their average PDI-scores (%).

Results

Periodontal Disease Index (PDI)

The majority of the recruits, who had all six of the teeth examined when using *Ramfjord's* index, exhibited serious lesions of gingivitis (Scores 3,1 to 4,0), (Fig. 6.4).

None of the subjects presented healthy periodontal conditions. In approximately 25% of the cases the gingival inflammation had already led to root exposure. Nearly all of the recruits had to be advised to seek periodontal treatment.

Gingival inflammation (Sulcus-Bleeding-Index, SBI)

Symptoms of varying degrees of inflammation were found in 98.5% of all recruits. Bleeding on probing of the gingival sulcus was considered the first sign of inflammation and was found in more than half of the subjects. Colour changes and bleeding following probing were determined in 35% of the recruits. Additional changes in structure were considered to be a sign of very severe inflammation (Scores 2,1 to 4,0) and these were found in 8.0% of the cases.

Plaque-Index (modified according to Quigley and Hein)

Over 75% of the subjects had moderate degrees of plaque formation (Scores 0,1 to 2,0 covering up to ¼ of the tooth surface). There were even greater amounts of plaque (Scores 2,1 to 4,0) in the remaining 25%.

Supragingival calculus

Most of the recruits (32.8%) had calculus ranging from 0.6 to 1.0 mm in extent. Only 3 recruits (2.2%) were free of calculus. Greater amounts of calculus (more than 1.0 mm) were seen in 57.5% of the subjects.

Pocket depths

No recruits exhibited a physiological sulcus depth of 1.0 mm or less. Pathological gingival pockets could be found in 18.9% of the subjects.

Radiological and dental findings

The results of the radiological analysis included location of missing teeth, determination of triangulations, radiologically visible calculus, overhanging restoration and crown margins, and determination of the distance from the cementoenamel junction to the alveolar crest.

In 43% of the subjects, all 24 tooth surfaces were present, in 42.2% 1 to 4 were missing and in 10.4% 5 to 8 tooth surfaces were missing. Three per cent were missing 9 to 12 surfaces, 0.7% were missing 13 to 16 surfaces and 0.7% were missing as many as 21 to 24 surfaces. Despite the age of the recruits (an average of 20.3 years), fewer than half still had all of the 6-year molars. In fact 3% had lost all four of the 6-year molars.

The term 'triangulation' is used to indicate initial bone loss, which occurs when inflammation reaches the alveolar crest. In the x-ray this bone loss is triangular in shape and is considered to be the first radiologically visible sign of periodontal bone loss. In 74.1% of the cases this condition could be definitely ruled out. Twenty-five per cent of the subjects exhibited triangulation on 1 to 4 tooth surfaces and, in a further 0.7%, 5 to 8 surfaces were involved.

In the process of identifying overhanging restorations and crowns, no subdivision was considered. The maximum number of surfaces, which had been restored by fillings or crowns, was 12 in all of the subjects examined. In 37.1% of the subjects, 1 to 4 surfaces were restored by fillings which did not have overhangs, whereas in 2.2% of the cases there were 5 to 12 surfaces without overhanging restorations. Overhanging restorations were found on 1 to 4 surfaces in 34.8% of all the cases and on 5 to 8 surfaces in 2.2%.

The investigation into dental habits, which was conducted simultaneously, showed that in comparison with similar studies of Swiss recruits, German recruits had a notably poorer awareness of health and poorer attitudes toward oral hygiene techniques.

The German recruits were more likely to wait until they had a toothache before consulting a dentist. They also presented poorer oral hygiene, ate snacks and smoked more frequently. The lack of knowledge regarding oral hygiene techniques and the level of oral hygiene among German soldiers were causes for concern.

The attitude towards the dentist was shown to be mainly negative. Almost half of the recruits visited a dentist solely for treatment of pain. Only about 20% made regular visits every 6 months to have their teeth examined. More than half of the subjects gave fear of pain as the reason for not seeing a dentist.

As was expected, most of the recruits knew very little about their own teeth and their function. Many considered 'periodontitis' to be equivalent to 'tooth decay' or an infectious disease. Only every third recruit connected the term 'periodontitis' with such conditions as gingival inflammation or periodontal disease. The function of the teeth in chewing was also unclear to the majority of the recruits. Some considered the anterior teeth to be more important than the posterior teeth. Almost half of them believed that the loss of teeth is inevitable with age. This fatalistic attitude was in contrast to the desire of 95% of the subjects to keep their teeth as long as possible.

The lack of education and information regarding the teeth, oral hygiene and the functions of the dentist was even more obvious when the recruits were questioned about the oral hygiene instructions they had received. Only about 5%, that is every twentieth subject, received specific instruction from his dentist, or assistant, in cleaning teeth. Seventy-five per cent did not say who taught them how to clean their teeth. Parents, who are actually the first people one should expect to teach the child to handle a toothbrush, were surprisingly seldom named as the instructors. Less than every fifth subject bought a new toothbrush every 3 months, 60%

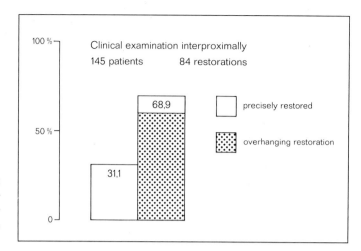

Fig. 6.5 Clinical findings in posterior teeth. Of 848 restorations, 584 (68,9%) have overhangs (35-year-olds, N = 145, Münster, 1981).

used each toothbrush for at least 6 months.

Most of the recruits only used a toothbrush in cleaning the teeth. Other aids were relatively unfamiliar to them. Every tenth subject claimed to use a water irrigant device regularly, every third used a toothpick. Since medical toothpicks were fairly unfamiliar, those used were generally sharpened matches.

Gingival bleeding was observed in 70% of the subjects to be the first visible clinical sign of gingivitis. Of these, every fifth subject had frequent episodes of bleeding. However, very few considered this gingival bleeding to be sufficient reason to see a dentist. The majority did nothing or took useless or improper measures, such as gargling or brushing less often.

Münster Study of 35-Year-Old Adults

One hundred and forty-five 35-year-old Münster residents were examined in 1981. The Periodontal-Treatment-Need-System[10, 22] was used as the standard measure. The classes were subdivided into groups 0, A, B and C according to the criteria of this index-system (Table 6.5):

This study was part of a joint investigation with the University of Zurich.[9, 11]

Results

Dental caries and restorations

The average number of DMF-teeth among the 35-year-old Münster residents was 18.2%. An average of almost 8 teeth had been restored and the same number had carious lesions. Table 6.6 compares the results of the Münster study and a similar study in Zurich.[14]

Table 6.5 Criteria for determining periodontal treatment needs according to *Johansen et al.*[22]

Group 0	no periodontal treatment required
Group A	motivation, oral hygiene instruction and polishing required
Group B	in addition to A, in one or more quadrants supra- and/or subgingival calculus removal and removal of iatrogenic irritants required
Group C	as in B, in addition in one or more quadrants periodontal pockets of more than 5 mm requiring a curettage or flap operation

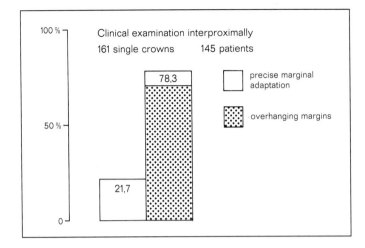

Fig. 6.6 Of 161 single crowns 36 (21,7%) can be judged clinically as having precise marginal adaptation (35-year-olds, N = 145, Münster, 1981).

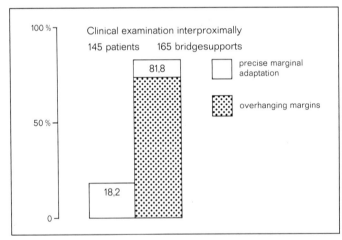

Fig. 6.7 Approximately 18% of all bridge supports show precise marginal adaptation (35-year-olds, N = 145, Münster, 1981).

A further part of the Münster study examined the condition of interproximal restorations. Of a total of 848 fillings, 69% had cervical overhangs (Fig. 6.5). A similar situation was found in relation to crowns. Of 161 single crowns, 78% were overhanging (Fig. 6.6), whereas among crowns serving as bridge abutments, 82% were overhanging (Fig. 6.7).

Subgingival restorations have a deleterious effect on the adjacent periodontal tissues, even when they appear to be clinically perfect in terms of surface and marginal adaptation. The standard of restorative treatment found in these studies will obviously contribute to further adverse iatrogenic influences on the periodontal tissues.

Periodontal disease

The assessment of periodontal treatment needs was of particular interest. The results obtained using the periodontal treatment need index of *Johansen et al.*[22] are presented on Table 6.5. There was no

Table 6.6 DMF-teeth among 35-year-old Münster and Zurich residents.

DMF-T	Münster	Zürich (*Fasler-Chu et al.* 1981)
carious	4,5	0,3
filled	7,8	16,0
filled/carious	3,4	1,3
missing	2,5	2,3
total	18,2	19,9

A comparison of the examination findings of other European cities (Table 6.7) showed that such treatment measures as were required by Group C were necessary for 47% of the subjects examined in Zurich, 37% in Oslo, and 82% in Poznan (Poland). It is necessary to emphasize that, in spite of the fact that periodontal treatment of a patient must be planned individually depending on the findings, motivation, cooperation etc., the PTNI is a reliable instrument for the assessment of treatment need.

case in Group 0 – 'no treatment required'. Acceptable periodontal conditions, for which motivation, instruction and polishing alone were indicated (Group A), were found in 7% of all subjects examined. 43% of all the 35-year-olds would have required a more intensive programme of scaling in addition to motivation and instruction (Group B). Approximately 50% fell into Group C, as several quadrants required a curettage or flap operation in addition to the other treatment measures (Table 6.7).

Dental behaviour and attitudes

Attitudes concerning oral hygiene habits and regimens were determined in a survey of the 35-year-old Münster residents (Table 6.8). Half of the subjects visited the dentists twice a year. The other half saw the dentist rarely or not at all. As regards the frequency of the dental visits, practically all of this kind of treatment falls into the category of so-called 'traditional care'. This care hardly makes it possible to maintain the periodontium in a healthy state.[3, 4, 5] It was found that nearly 80% no-

Table 6.7 Periodontal treatment needs according to PTN-System.

Group	Treatment required	Münster N = 145 %	Zürich N = 159 (*Meier et al.* 1979) %	Oslo N = 117 (*Hansen* and *Johansen* 1977) %	Poznan N = 25 (*Wierzbicka et al.* 1977) %
0	none	0,0	8,8	1,7	0,0
A	Motivation Oral Hygiene instruction	6,9	7,0	7,7	0,0
B	Overhang and Calculus Removal	43,0	37,1	53,0	18,0
C	Surgical pocket elimination (curettage, flap)	50,1	47,1	37,6	82,0
Total		100,0	100,0	100,0	100,0

Table 6.8 Percentage Distribution of the various possible answers to five questions, which reflect the attitudes concerning oral hygiene and the level of understanding among 145 35-year-old Münster residents.

How often do you visit the dentist?	twice a year	51,7%
	once a year	27,6% } 79,3%
	every two years	15,2%
	never	5,5%
Do your gums bleed when you clean your teeth?	often	8,3%
	sometimes	69,0%
	never	20,7%
	no answer	2,0%
Did anyone ever show you how to thoroughly clean your teeth?	yes	32,7%
	no	67,3%
What other oral hygiene aids do you use regularly?	none	60,7%
	dental floss	4,1%
	Waterpik	28,3%
	medical toothpicks	10,3%
	magnifying mirror	1,4%
	(several answers possible)	
Do you know the causes of bleeding of the gums and gum recession?	definitely yes	12,4%
	vaguely	57,9%
	no	29,7%
Do you believe that information concerning tooth and gum care would be of value to you?	yes	82,1%
	no	4,8%
	no opinion	9,0%
	no answer	4,1%

ticed the symptom of 'bleeding gums' but they were less informed about the cause of the disease. Only 32% stated that they had received thorough instructions concerning cleaning of the teeth. Of this group only half had been instructed by professionals (i.e. dentist, dental assistant or dental hygienist). Only a small percentage were familiar with oral hygiene aids or used these correctly. There is a definite need to market dental care items. Sixty per cent of those questioned were not familiar with any tooth care aids. If dental floss and medical toothpicks are only rarely used, interproximal oral hygiene is virtually non-existent.

Conclusion and Summary

If one analyzes the results of these studies, one comes to the conclusion that the oral hygiene, as well as the periodontal conditions of the population in the various age groups surveyed, are extremely poor and there is a need for systematic periodontal treatment for all age groups. A survey conducted by the WHO shows periodontal disease to be one of the most widespread diseases of mankind. Periodontal disease is progressive in nature. Gingivitis develops into marginal periodontitis, which attacks the deeper areas of the supporting structure and leads to bone resorption and development of pockets. As a rule, the disease process becomes more serious when the patient is over 20 years of age and the majority of the cases are chronic.

If we conclude from our epidemiological findings that the frequency of periodontal diseases in adults is equal to or greater than the caries incidence, then the same degree of attention and dental service should be devoted to the prophylaxis and therapy for periodontal diseases as is devoted to the treatment of caries. If one considers that the systematic treatment of periodontal disease comprises only approximately 1% of all dental treatments, then that means that on average only two or three systematic periodontal treatment cases per year are performed in each dental office in the Federal Republic of Germany. The curative practice of dentistry has at least reached a turning point for the areas of caries and periodontal diseases. It is evident that dental caries and periodontal disease cannot be controlled using reparative and restorative measures. The average working hours of a dentist do not suffice to deal with the increased need which he creates through his restorative services. As we were able to show in our epidemiological study, the situation in the areas of restoration and crown therapy among 35-year-olds is extremely unfavorable. Every restoration, every crown is only an incomplete substitute for the natural tooth and generally either promotes or aggravates periodontal diseases.

References

1. Anagnou-Vareldzides A., Tsamin A., Zervogianes D. and Mitsis F. I.
   Oral hygiene and gingival health in Greek airforce cadet candidates. Community Dent. Oral Epidemiol., 1982, 10: 60–65.

2. Arno A., Waerhaug J., Lövdal A. and Schei O.
   Incidence of gingivitis as related to sex, occupation, tobacco consumption, toothbrushing and age. Oral Surg., 1958, 11: 587–595.

3. Axelsson P. and Lindhe J.
   The effect of a preventive programme on dental plaque, gingivitis and caries in schoolchildren. Results after one and two years. J. Clin. Periodontol., 1974, 1: 126–138.

4. Axelsson P. and Lindhe J.
   Effect of controlled oral hygiene procedures on caries and periodontal disease in adults. J. Clin. Periodontol., 1978, 5: 133–151.

5. Axelsson P. and Lindhe J.
   The significance of maintenance care in the treatment of periodontal disease. J. Clin. Periodontol., 1981, 8: 281–294.

6. Bayirli G. S. and Curilović Z.
   Periodontal condition in Turkish recruits. Community Dent. Oral Epidemiol., 1976, 4: 25–29.

7. Bayirli G. S. and Curilović Z.
   Periodontal condition in Turkish recruits. Community Dent. Oral Epidemiol., 1979, 7: 57–64.

8. Brandtzaeg P. and Jameson H. C.
   A study of periodontal health and oral hygiene in Norwegian army recruits. J. Periodontol., 1964, 35: 302–307.

9. Carstens S.
   Mundhygieneverhalten, Mundhygiene- und Parodontalzustand bei 35jährigen einer deutschen Großstadt. Thesis Medical Faculty, Univ. of Münster, West Germany, 1984.

10. Curilović Z.
    Parodontalzustand bei einer Gruppe von Schweizer Rekruten. Schweiz. Monatsschr. Zahnheilkd., 1972, 82: 437–451.

11. Curilović Z.
    Epidemiologische Daten der Parodontalerkrankungen in der Bundesrepublik Deutschland. Swiss Dent., 1982, 3: 63–69.

12. Demitriou N. A.
    Epidemiologic research of parodontopathies in a group of 2.564 Greek males, 21-years-old. J. West Soc. Periodontol., 1966, 14: 93–94.

13. Engelberger B. and Rateitschak K. H.
    Parodontaler Knochenschwund und Kariesbefall bei Erwachsenen. Schweiz. Monatsschr. Zahnheilkd., 1970, 80: 1295–1310.

14. Fasler-Chu B. B., Curilović Z., Wally M., Ottiker J. and Meier Ch.
    Zahnverlust und Zahnersatz bei einer Gruppe 35jähriger Zürcher. Schweiz. Monatsschr. Zahnheilkd., 1981, 91: 166.

15. Germann M. A., Curilović Z., Sayer U. P. and Renggli H. H.
    Parodontalzustand bei einer Gruppe von Schwei-

zer Rekruten – Röntgenologische Befunde. Schweiz. Monatsschr. Zahnheilkd., 1973, 83: 1220–1229.

16. *Gjermo P.*
International bite wing survey (1979–1980). Proceedings FDI, Hamburg, 1980.

17. *Goh S. W.* and *Wong M. O.*
The prevalence of materia alba, calculus deposites and periodontal disease in Singapore School children. Dent. J. Malaisia Singapore, 1983, 13: 3–10.

18. *Gülzow H.-J.*
Über Zahn- und Mundpflegegewohnheiten von Studierenden der Universität Erlangen-Nürnberg. Dtsch. zahnärztl. Z., 1971, 26: 9.

19. *Hansen B. F.* and *Johansen J. R.*
Periodontal treatment needs of 35-year-old citizens in Oslo. J. Clin. Periodontol., 1977, 4: 263–271.

20. *Hansen B. F., Gjermo P.* and *Bellini H. T.*
A multinational study on the prevalence of radiographic bone loss in young adults. Community Dent. Oral Epidemiol., 1984 (in press).

21. *Holland-Moritz R.*
Zahnpflegegewohnheiten – Mund- und Gebißbefunde – eine vergleichende Untersuchung an Soldaten der Bundeswehr. Zahnärztl. Mitt. 1975, 62: 1049–1052.

22. *Johansen J. R., Gjermo P.* and *Bellini H. T.*
A system to classify the need for periodontal treatment. Acta Odontol. Scand., 1973, 31: 297.

23. *Jorkjend L.* and *Birkeland J. M.*
Plaque and gingivitis among Norwegian children participating in a dental health program. Community Dent. Oral Epidemiol., 1973, 1: 41–46.

24. *Lange D. E.*
Epidemiologische Untersuchungen über das Vorkommen und die Häufigkeit von Parodontopathien in ausgewählten Altersgruppen in der Bundesrepublik Deutschland. Öster. Z. Stomatol., 1982, 79: 307.

25. *Lange D. E.* and *Peric B.*
Röntgenologische und klinische Untersuchungen an ersten Molaren von 15- und 16jährigen zur Frühdiagnostik der Parodontopathien. Dtsch. zahnärztl. Z., 1981, 36: 449–450.

26. *Lange D. E.* and *Schwöppe G.*
Epidemiologische Untersuchungen an Rekruten der Bundeswehr (Mund- und Gebißbefunde). Dtsch. zahnärztl. Z., 1981, 36: 432–434.

27. *Lennon M. A.* and *Davis R. M.*
Prevalence and distribution of alveolar bone loss in a population of 15-year-old schoolchildren. J. Clin. Periodontol., 1974, 1: 175–182.

28. *Lighthner L. M., O'Leary T. J., Dranke R. B., Crump P. P., Jividen G. J.* and *Junghans J. A.*
The periodontal status of incoming Air Force Academy cadets. J. Amer. Dent. Assoc., 1967, 72: 111–117.

29. *Löe H.*
Dynamik der Entwicklung und Progression der parodontalen Läsionen. Dtsch. zahnärztl. Z., 1982, 37: 533–539.

30. *Löe H., Theilade E.* and *Jensen S. B.*
Experimental gingivitis in man. J. Periodontol., 1965, 36: 177–187.

31. *Löe H., Anerud A., Boysen H.* and *Smith M.*
The natural history of periodontal disease in man. Study design and baseline data. J. Periodontal. Res., 1978 a, 13: 550–562.

32. *Löe H., Anerud A., Boysen H.* and *Smith M.*
The natural history of periodontal disease in man. The rate of periodontal destruction before 40 years of age. J. Periodontol., 1978 b, 49: 607–620.

33. *Löe H., Anerud A., Boysen H.* and *Smith M.*
The natural history of periodontal disease in man. Tooth mortality rates before 40 years of age. J. Periodontal. Res., 1978 c, 13: 563–572.

34. *Lutz F., Curilović J., Renggli H. H., Saxer U.-P., Schmid M. O., Berchtold H.* and *Bandi A.*
Orale Gesundheit für jedermann – ein unerreichbares Ziel? Analyse einer Umfragung bei 1200 Schweizer Rekruten. Schweiz. Monatsschr. Zahnheilkd., 1977, 87: 633–647.

35. *Mann J., Cormier P. P., Green P., Ram C. A., Miller M. F.* and *Ship I. I.*
Loss of periodontal attachment in adolescents. Community Dent. Oral Epidemiol., 1981, 9: 135–141.

36. *Marthaler T. M.*
Epidemiologie von Zahnkaries, Gingivitis und Zahnstein bei 7646 Schweizer Schulkindern. Schweiz. Monatsschr. Zahnheilkd., 1968, 78: 19–35.

37. *Meier Ch., Curilović Z., Wally M., Chu B. B.* and *Ottiker J.*
Parodontalbehandlungsnotwendigkeit, Motivation und Informationsstand bei einer Gruppe 35jähriger Züricher. Schweiz. Monatsschr. Zahnheilkd., 1979, 89: 699–711.

38. *Metha F. S., Sanjana M. K.* and *Shroff B. C.*
Prevalence of periodontal disease. 5. Epidemiology in Indian child population in relation to their periodontal status. Int. Dent. J., 1956, 6: 31–40.

39. *Mobley E.* and *Smith S. H.*
Some social and economic factors relating to periodontal disease among young Negroes. J. Amer. Dent. Assoc., 1963, 66: 486–491.

40. *Perić B.*
Klinische und röntgenologische Untersuchungen über das Vorkommen und die Häufigkeit von juvenilen Parodontopathien (ein Beitrag zur Früherkennung von Parodontopathien). Thesis Medical Faculty, Univ. of Münster West-Germany, 1983.

41. *Quigley G.* and *Hein J.*
Comparative cleansing efficiency of manual and power brushing. J. Amer. Dent. Assoc., 1962, 65: 26–29.

42. *Ramfjord A.*
Indices for prevalence and incidence of periodontal disease. J. Periodontol., 1959, 30: 51–59.

43. *Russell A. L.*
A system of classification and scoring of prevalence surveys of periodontal disease. J. Dent. Res., 1956. 35: 350–359.

44. *Russell A. L.*
A social factor associated with the severity of periodontal disease. J. Dent. Res., 1957, 36: 922–926.

45. *Russell A. L.*
Some epidemiological characteristics of periodontal disease in a series of urban populations. J. Periodontol., 1957, 28: 286–293.

46. *Russell A. L.*
Epidemiology of periodontal disease. Int. Dent. J., 1967, 17: 282–296.

47. *Samuelson G., Grahnen H.* and *Lindström G.*
An epidemiological study of child health and nutrition in a northern Swedish county. V. Oral health studies. Odontol. Revy. Lund., 1971, 22: 189–220.

48. *Saxer U. P., Curilović Z., Germann M. A.* and *Renggli H. H.*
Mundpflegegewohnheiten bei einer Gruppe von Schweizer Rekruten. Schweiz. Monatsschr. Zahnheilkd., 1972, 82: 1090–1099.

49. *Sheiham A.*
Dental cleanliness and chronic periodontal disease. Studies on populations in Britain. Brit. Dent. J., 1970, 129: 413–418.

50. *Suomi J. D.*
Periodontal disease and oral hygiene in institutionalized populations. Report of an epidemiological study. J. Periodontol., 1969, 40: 5–10.

51. *Suomi J. D.* and *Doyle J.*
Oral hygiene and periodontal disease in an adult population in the United States. J. Periodontol., 1972, 43: 677–681.

52. *Schei O., Waerhaug J., Lövdal A.* and *Arno A.*
Alveolar bone loss as related to hygiene and age. J. Periodontol., 1959, 30: 7–16.

52. *Schiffner D., Maier R.* and *Franz G.*
Untersuchung über das Mundhygieneverhalten verschiedener sozialer Gruppen in der Bundesrepublik Deutschland und in Hamburg. Kariesprophylaxe, 1982, 4: 64–70.

54. *Schönauer T.* and *Godt H.*
Über das Mundhygienebewußtsein schwedischer und deutscher Schulkinder. Dtsch. zahnärztl. Z., 1975, 30: 795.

55. *Schuh E., Fischer R., Holler G., Hackl P.* and *Moser F.*
Der Zahn- und Parodontalzustand von Schulkindern in Österreich. Quintessenz, 1981, Ref. 6225: 939–945.

56. *Schwöppe G.*
Epidemiologische Untersuchungen an einer Gruppe von Rekruten der Bundeswehr (Mund- und Gebißbefunde, Mundhygienezustand, Zahnpflegegewohnheiten). Thesis Medical Faculty, Univ. of Münster, West-Germany, 1979.

57. *Schwöppe G.* and *Lange D. E.*
Mundhygienezustand und Zahnpflegegewohnheiten von Rekruten der Bundeswehr. Dtsch. zahnärztl. Z., 1981, 36: 429–431.

58. *Tan H. H., Ter Horst G.* and *Kekking Y. M.*
Dental knowledge, attitude and behavior in 12-year-old Dutch suburban children. Community Dent. Oral Epidemiol., 1981, 9: 122–127.

59. *Wierzbicka M., Limanowska H., Stopa J.* and *Jwanicka E.*
Beurteilung der Behandlungsbedürftigkeit bei Parodontalerkrankungen mit dem Bellini-System. Stoma. DDR, 1977, 27: 610.

60. *Wingerath H.-D.*
Mundhygieneverhalten von 14- und 15jährigen Schülern im Raum Bottrop unter soziologischen Gesichtspunkten. Thesis Medical Faculty, Univ. of Münster, West-Germany, 1980.

61. *Wingerath H.-D.* and *Lange D. E.*
Mundhygieneverhalten von 14- und 15jährigen Schülern unter soziologischen Gesichtspunkten. Dtsch. zahnärztl. Z., 1982, 37: 565–568.

62. World Health Organization. Epidemiology, etiology and prevention of periodontal diseases. Technical report series 621, WHO Geneva, 1978.

7. The Influence of Oral Health Delivery Systems on the Awareness and Prevalence of Periodontal Breakdown in the Belgian Population

Daniel van Steenberghe

Introduction

Although definitely belonging to the industrialized countries with a very high standard of living (283.000 BF/per capita per year)[11] and extensive dental treatment facilities, Belgium has a rather different profile concerning periodontal treatment than other Northern EEC countries. Therefore, it would seem to be an interesting model to use in order to evaluate the effects of public health facilities, which are clearly not periodontally-oriented, on the periodontal condition and treatment possibilities for the population. It will also be of assistance in formulating recommendations for future policy.

Prevalence of Periodontal Disease in Belgium

A major problem in the evaluation of the periodontal problem is the lack of any significant epidemiological surveys concerning oral health in Belgium. The few studies published, concerning caries incidence and/or tooth loss, do not correspond to standard requirements for epidemiological investigations. A scientific approach has been applied in surveys presently in progress in some universities.

Only preliminary data are available of the retrospective part of one of these studies concerning the degree of interproximal bone loss and missing teeth, evaluated by orthopantomograms using the methodology described by *Björn* and *Holmberg*.[5] A transparent ruler is used to evaluate bone height as a fraction of the total tooth length, since it is often impossible on radiographs to determine the cemento-enamel junction. The quoted authors demonstrated that bone height measurements on orthopantomograms are valuable for mass screening. The presently reported results originate from 264 orthopantomograms, out of a series of 1.000, taken on patients who visited the department of oral surgery. Their social status, educational level and area of origin showed a great variety. Most of them were sent to the department by their dentist, their physician or another department within the academic clinic, for such reasons as extraction of wisdom teeth, bone pathology, fractures, detection of intraoral focal infection, etc. Their oral health status and motivation for seeking dental treatment was therefore rather representative of the population. Further details of the methodology and of an ongoing prospective study on a representative group of the population is reported later.[7, 12]

The distribution of alveolar bone loss within the dentition, taking into consideration the age group, is shown in Fig. 7.1, while in Fig. 7.2 the loss of two teeth is present-

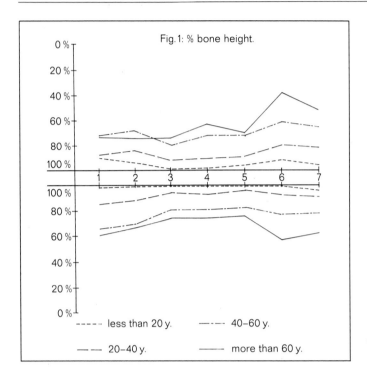

Fig. 7.1 Bone height (%) within the dentition according to age groups.

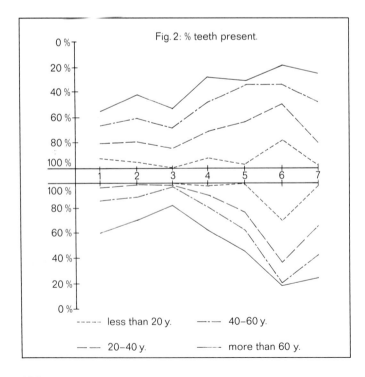

Fig. 7.2 Teeth (%) present within the dentition according to age groups.

Table 7.1 Frequency distribution of marginal fit of premolar – molar restorations and of alveolar bone loss.

		No bone loss	< 25%	> 25%
< 30 y	No filling	82.2	17.6	0.3
	Well-adapted	75.5	20.6	1.0
	Overhang	67.4	27.4	5.3
30–50 y	No filling	43.5	43.4	13.1
	Well-adapted	48.0	44.4	7.6
	Overhang	29.3	54.6	16.1
> 50 y	No filling	19.2	45.7	35.1
	Well-adapted	33.0	55.7	11.3
	Overhang	12.7	53.1	34.2

ed in a similar manner. The parallelisms between the curves is striking. Although no causal relationship can be put forward, it could be interpreted that periodontal breakdown was responsible for an important proportion of tooth extractions. This distribution within the oral cavity is in accordance with other epidemiological data available, but the loss of attachment is quite important in the young Belgian population, when compared with other industrialized countries.[9] Although the later authors measured loss of attachment clinically, one can extrapolate the present radiological data to enable a certain comparison.

It is impossible to discriminate between periodontal pathology, caries incidence and forceps level when interpreting figures concerning tooth loss in the population. No significant data are available concerning edentulousness in the Belgian population. Calculus was detected on 25% of the readable surfaces in the whole dentition.

The number of restorations in the remaining dentition gives an idea of the oral consciousness of the sample studied. On the 2526 premolar and molar teeth evaluated, 869 had either a metal restoration or a crown. Only 15.8% of the approximal surfaces were restored, which contrasts with the 50% reported by *Björn, Björn* and *Grkovic*[4] for dental-conscious inhabitants of the Malmö area. In the presently reported survey, the quality of marginal fit of metal restorations was also examined in the premolar – molar region to evaluate a possible relationship with bone loss. It is evident that on orthopantomograms only gross overhangs or underfillings can be seen. Therefore intraoral radiographs would give an even higher figure for defective restorations.[4] As can be seen in Table 7.1, a clear interaction exists between overt overhangs, or underfillings, and approximal bone loss.

Other indications of the periodontal aspects of the Belgian population can be found in the lack of use of interdental aids for plaque control. Of some 2.000 patients who visited the department of periodontology at the Catholic University of Leuven, presenting a rather equal distribution of rural and town area origins, none had daily practice in the use of either tooth picks or floss for at least one year. Those patients who had resided in foreign countries, or who had contacted a foreign dentist or oral hygienist were disregarded. Few patients had been instructed adequately by their dentists in approximal plaque-control. One of two tooth picks available on the Belgian market sold 35.000 tooth picks per month in 1980, but some 100.000 per month in 1982. These figures indicate a rapid increase, but an incredibly low use. The use of floss is even more sporadic in the country, but is increasing rapidly too. The indices for selling were in 1978: 100, 1979: 170, 1980: 220, 1981: 350. The frequency of toothbrushing is also below average (one tooth brush sold for every 3 persons per year, and less than 200 g of tooth paste per capita sold per year).

Although the data available are very limited, it is apparent that periodontal breakdown has a high incidence and the periodontal consciousness of the population nearly nonexistant. For a few years however, a rapid increase has been apparent. Several explanations for this are set out below.

Existing Oral Health Care

Education

In Belgium, dentistry has been taught at the universities since 1929. It has been a 5 year curriculum, with the 3 first years common with medicine. Since 1972 a separate curriculum has been started, 2 candidatures and 3 licence years, although the teaching during the first 2 years has a broad common base with medicine. The preclinical and clinical teaching during the 3 licence years is comparable to other EEC countries. However, in the whole curriculum, skilfulness and technical aspects are more stressed than biological thinking or treatment planning. This is of course very detrimental to periodontal thinking and practice. Too often the student is evaluated on the technical qualities of an isolated performance, rather than on the judiciousness of a global patient treatment. Recently, a person with responsibility for study advice, at one of the universities, wrote that students in dentistry often doubted in their choice between dentistry and 'other academic studies which have hardly any relationship with dentistry, such as medicine, veterinary medicine and biology . . . while training for dental technician is probably more close to dentistry'.[8]

Periodontology has been taught intensively for only a few years at some universities, while others still lack a well-defined training. Mostly, periodontology is started during the last, or 2 final, years of the curriculum. The influence of introducing periodontology into dental education, and also of some postgraduate teaching, gave rise to changes in the consciousness of the dental profession. Of course it will take many more years before this will lead to a change of attitude on a large scale. Some indications are encouraging. While some 5 years ago, periodontal probes were not known by most dentists, presently, at most universities, all students buy them with the rest of their clinical equipment. Their use after leaving university remains however unevaluated. The important fact is that during the last 2 years some 30.000 leaflets, which dentists can buy to inform their patients about periodontitis, have been sold. A Society of Periodontology was started in 1981, and its scientific meetings are regularly attended by more than 200 members.

Little attention is being paid towards motivation techniques, patient-dentist relations, community aspects of the profession, and epidemiology. It is evident that this results in a poor motivation for the student to start preventive periodontal treatment.

A little more than five trained periodontologists are presently practicing in the country, while a few more dentists or oral surgeons claim a periodontally-orientated practice. There is no officially recognized specialization, except at one university where dentists obtain a university diploma of specialist in periodontology after a 3 years full-time training (reduced to 2 years for oral surgeons). However, similar training programmes are present at some other universities. This means that the patients are unable to distinguish between the trained periodontologists and those who are not. This leads unhappily to abuses, such as surgical pocket elimination without proper plaque control, or routine placement of free gingival grafts for recessions. The lack of periodontologists and of their recognition are two major problems in Belgium, which will increase with the rapidly increasing demand for treatment. The latter is a logical consequence of an increasing consciousness of the periodontal problem by the medical professions and the population as a whole.

Until now, oral hygienists cannot practice in the country, and their introduction is at present being opposed by some representatives of the dental profession. The main problem seems to be the fear of a plethora of dentists (see below) and/or a vaguely defined framework for the future oral hygienists. In the latter matter, Belgium has a tendency to follow other latin countries, instead of the Northern part of the EEC. It is evidently a waste of resources to have a university trained practitioner undertake plaque control.[14] The result is that patients mostly receive no oral hygiene instructions in dental practice (see p. 102). In some schools, some uncoordinated positive efforts are being made by untrained volunteer dentists, dental students and even social assistants. The results are not being evaluated, but several reports have indicated that the roll technique is still taught by some, and that motivation is exclusively oriented toward caries prevention, including eating of hard food. This means that, for the mo-

ment, trained manpower is nearly nonexistant for either the preventive or curative treatment of periodontal disease, although a high dentist/population ratio has been obtained.

Manpower

More and more people seem concerned with having too many dentists in the population in the future. In fact, the dentist/population ratio in 1982 was about 1/2.100. However in 1962 the ratio was 1/5.000 and in 1972 1/3.800.[10] Because of a sensibly declining student population for a few years, further increase is not so steep, though still significant. This means that already, more than half of the dentist population is under 35 years of age. Increasing financial problems arise for more and more dentists, since the demand from the population has not followed the dramatic increase in the number of practitioners. It has not been apparent until now that, because of their decreasing frequency of patients per dentist, the latter devoted more time to preventive or curative periodontal treatment. Lack of training, unavailable social security reimbursements for periodontal treatment might be a partial explanation. As in other countries, there might be an increasing fear of overtreatment in the restorative field of the patients seeking oral care. One could hope that, with the young age of the dentist population, a change of postgraduate training in a more periodontal and preventive oriented direction might occur, but possibilities are limited for the present.

Social security

Belgium has extensive medical care reimbursements for all employed people, regardless of age or income. Independent workers and their families benefit a more limited reimbursement (only x-rays and surgical treatment). Anyone is free to visit any physician or dentist he wants. The latter will give him a formulary for the fixed reimbursement. This freedom enchances the consultation of several practitioners, or of a specialist, without having to refer to the general practitioner. Generally for dental treatment, 75% of the official honorarium is reimbursed, but the dentist is partially free to ask more. For x-rays or surgical procedures, 100% is refunded. No reimbursement exists for fixed prosthetic rehabilitation, or for any prosthetic work below the age of 50. For older people, some reimbursement exists for removable prostheses when enough opposing teeth are missing. No reimbursement whatsoever exists for periodontal therapy, except for a very small honorarium for gingivectomy. This means that patients will not receive a formulary after all preventive and most curative periodontal treatments, with the evident negative reactions which can discourage some practitioners to start or continue this kind of treatment. On the other hand, the same is true for crown and bridge work, where this problem is more easily resolved because of an established tradition with both the dentist and the patient.

The discrimination against periodontal treatment, and preventive measures in general, in this extensive social security system is damaging to the patient's dental and periodontal health.

The lack of quality control (which theoretically exists for endodontic treatment) concerning marginal fit of restorative work also has negative influences on the periodontal condition of the population (see above).

Since no compulsory regular controls by the dentist exist, a high percentage of the population never or hardly ever visits the dentist. The result is that no financial incentive exists for prevention and often the only treatment will be subtotal or total extraction of the remaining teeth.

Reimbursement for dental treatments represents less than 5% of the total security funds, which means 4 to 5 billion Belgian Francs.

Public health organizations

All administrative functions concerning oral health, either at the Ministry of Health, the Academy of Medicine, Red Cross, etc., are occupied by physicians who mostly do not have a diploma in dentistry. Because of the resulting lack of knowledge and interest concerning the field, no important initiatives have ever been taken to promote oral health. In schools, dental examination is either nonexistant or performed in a very limited number by volunteering dentists or supervised dental students. Since oral hygienists are unavailable, preventive measures cannot be taken on a large scale (see above). The Ministry of Education also does not have an organized programme to offer the students some elementary information concerning oral health. Since information concerning dental and periodontal disease is rare in the media, the immense majority of the population is unaware of periodontal pathologies and of their cause. For example, less than 1% of the 2.000 patients who were referred to our periodontal department or visited it directly, were aware that plaque can cause gingival inflammation.

Scientific organizations in the dental field have recently taken some initiatives to fill the existing gap. Lack of coordination or money give them a rather low profile.

Goal Formulations

It is evident from the abovementioned facts and data, that building up a framework with high level university education, high dentist/population ratios, extensive social security facilities do not lead to an acceptable level of oral health in an industrialized country with a very high standard of living.

Dentists, with a proper training in periodontology are needed to be able to diagnose periodontal diseases and be capable of setting up proper treatment or knowing when the patient has to be referred to a specialist. Since economic and social environment is becoming more and more similar in the EEC, and since medical profession are free to establish themselves in any of the member countries, a common university education programme should be established. It should not try to find the largest common denominator, but be oriented to the goals and future needs of the dental profession. This means that one should take into consideration the important decrease of caries frequency in most countries, which will increase the need for periodontal treatment,[2] the introduction of auxiliaries and a decreasing amount of money available both in social security systems and for potential patients. The periodontal aspects of dental treatments, such as orthodontics, extractions and especially restorative work, should receive ample attention in their respective fields. The student should be trained from the beginning in establishing a global treatment plan which corresponds to the goal of his professional education 'to maintain a healthy natural functioning dentition for life',[13] instead of in isolated technical skill. This means more emphasis on the biological basic sciences, an integrated clinical training and team approach, with preventive treatment from the first day.[6] If the latter is only added at the end of the curriculum, bad habits will already have developed which will be hard to change. Medical students should also be provided with adequate teaching in periodontal diseases and their interaction with systemic diseases.

The too rapid increase in dental manpower, while the populations demand is still very low, demonstrates the need for a governmental policy to let the number of students keep pace with that demand. The latter should of course be strongly stimulated towards acceptable levels. More outcomes should also be offered to the dentists, such as specialization, administrative and decision-making positions, scientific research, instead of discriminating them towards the physicians. The latter aspects will inevitably influence further decision-making by the government.

The need for a recognizable specialist in periodontology is evident, since one of the pathologies he is dealing with is more frequent than that of other already recognized specialities, such as orthodontics or oral surgery, and needs a long training to evaluate the possibilities and limitations of curative treatments in advanced cases. Several modalities concerning the exclusiveness of that speciality are possible. There is however a danger that a general practitioner may be reluctant to refer a patient to a colleague who will not seem different to the patient, as this can induce a loss of confidence and finally the loss of the patient. An acceleration of specialist training in periodontology is needed and postgraduate training of previously graduated dentists to familiarize them with routine preventive and surgical procedures. If one wants to have periodontal treatment on a large scale, most of the work will have to be performed by the general practitioners.

It is unnecessary to point out the necessity of oral hygienists in the public health system. Especially in the present economic situation, it is unthinkable to have prevention programmes performed on large numbers of the population by highly skilled dentists. It is a waste of money and educational investment, without even the certainty that the motivation for some of the more ancillary aspects of these programmes will be high. This was one of the policy statements at the EEC workshop in Dublin. The freedom of the establishment in any EEC country should be applied to them.

To influence the policy-makers, clear epidemiological data must be collected as soon as possible, and the impact on the population's health and on direct and indirect (nonattendance at work) financial costs underlined. It is evident that new goals should be put forward on the reimbursement policy of the social security system; more emphasis should be given to preventive and periodontal treatments, with restrictions to the frequency of treatment and the qualification of the practitioner/auxiliary. If no reimbursement is available for preventive measures (instruction, scaling and root planing) the need for numerous oral hygienists will be even more evident. Of course, further pressure and 'lobbying' will be necessary to answer the needs, even if they are clearly demonstrated by epidemiologial data. The professional organizations could play a positive role in this effort.

Regular visits to the dentist could be made compulsory in the framework of the insurance system. The patient would keep the freedom of non-treatment, but would lose the right for reimbursement. These regular visits would allow screening of the periodontal susceptible individuals – and of caries – who would be forwarded to a more intense programme. As long as periodontal breakdown would not be detected beyond a certain index, the patients would be left in the general system. This kind of selection would reduce the costs of treatment sensibly, and would correspond to the present scientific approach of periodontal inflammation.

Public health organizations should stress the periodontal aspects of oral health, and take advice from scientific authorities before organizing actions or publishing information leaflets. Contradictory information is very demotivating. It is evident from many studies that preventive efforts should involve the whole community,[3] while school-based health education programmes should be integrated with other health instructions.

Media should be involved in public education, using well-known or leading people on a frequent basis. Cooperation with industries in the field could help to finance these projects.

Conclusion

It is evident that building up a costly educational and social security system does not sensibly benefit the oral health of the population as long as periodontal aspects are forgotten. A proper training of all dentists, the availability of more qualified periodontologists and oral hygienists, a balanced and more preventive-oriented reimbursement system, a compulsory screening system and large-scale information on the needs of the whole population will correspond to the final goals of oral health and of the dental profession.

References

1. *Agerbaek N.*
   Effect of regular small group instruction per se on oral health status of Danish schoolchildren. Community Dent. Oral Epidemiol., 1979, 7: 17–23.

2. *Ainamo J.*
   Significance of periodontal disease in Society. In Efficacy of Treatment Procedures in Periodontics. (Shanley D., ed.) Quintessence Books, Chicago 1980, pp. 299–312.

3. *Axelsson P.* and *Lindhe J.*
   Effect of controlled oral hygiene procedures on caries and periodontal disease in adults. J. Clin. Periodontol., 1978, 5: 133–151.

4. *Björn H.* and *Holmberg K.*
   Radiographic determination of periodontal bone destruction in epidemiological research. Odontol. Revy., 1966, 17: 232–250.

5. *Björn A. L., Björn H.* and *Grkovic B.*
   Marginal fit of restorations and its relation to periodontal bone level. Part I: Metal fillings. Odontol. Revy., 1969, 20: 311–321.

6. *Frandsen A.*
   Educational objectives in relation to provision of care. In Efficacy of Treatment Procedures in Peri-

odontics. (Shanley D. ed.) Quintessence books, Chicago, 1980, pp. 257–266.

7. *Gooris A., Quirynen M.* and *Steenberghe D. van.*
Iatrogenic factors influencing periodontal bone loss: a radiographic survey. 1984 (submitted).

8. *Hoornaert J.*
Tandheelkunde als beroepsuitweg. Dienst voor Studie-advies. Katholieke Universiteit Leuven, 1983, p. 3.

9. *Löe H., Anerud A., Boysen H.* and *Smith M.*
The natural history of periodontal disease in man. J. Periodontol., 1978, 49: 607–620.

10. Ministry of health, Brussels: Statistical report, 1981.

11. National Institute of Statistics. Brussels. Personal communication.

12. *Quirynen M., Gooris A.* and *Steenberghe D. van.*
Cross-classified categorical data analysis of the intra-oral distribution of periodontal bone loss in the Belgian population. 1984 (submitted).

13. *Sheiham A.*
An evaluation of the success of dental care in the United Kingdom. Brit. Dent. J., 1973, 135: 271–279.

14. *Waerhaug J.*
What is the objective of treatment: disease elimination, control or reduction? In Efficacy of Treatment Procedures in Periodontics. (Shanley D. ed.) Quintessence, Chicago, 1980, pp. 235–239.

8. Periodontal Disease and the Influence of Socio-Educational Factors in Adolescents

Diarmuid B. Shanley and Frances M. Ahern

Introduction

A Workshop was held in 1979 to consider the *Efficacy of Treatment Procedures in Periodontics*.[12] Concern was expressed about directing limited resources towards increasingly sophisticated procedures with little improvement in the general periodontal health levels of the community. It was stated that no major disease had ever been eradicated by treatment alone.[5] Emphasis was placed on setting objectives in patient care, such as the maintenance of a comfortable and functioning dentition for a lifetime by reducing the rate of periodontal destruction in many rather than seeking its total elimination in a few patients.[11] It was thought that such objectives might be achieved through community health education and care programmes. Social, educational and cultural factors constituted significant influences on the success of such an approach.[13]

McGreil[9] said that education, occupation and economic security are largely determined by social class position. This can influence a person's world view, his wants and aspirations. Oral and dental diseases have also been found to reflect the life styles of individuals. *Kiyak* found that important cultural differences exist in dental behaviour and were found to be related to knowledge and motives.[7] In a study on the *Demand and Need for Dental Care*, *Bulman et al*[3] showed a strong relationship between social strata and oral disease and that while the rules of dental health were known they were not practiced. The influence of social and educational factors have been shown to have a fundamental effect on dental care, oral health, perception and behaviour in oral health exercises.[2, 3, 10, 14, 15, 16]

The purpose of this study was to identify levels of dental disease in 15–17-year-old Dublin adolescents and to determine the influence of socio-educational factors on these findings. A questionnaire was also completed to determine their stated attitudes, behaviour and perception in relation to dental health, with the intention of relating these responses to the clinical findings and social groupings. Detailed analysis of inter-relationships between groups of questions and the clinical findings requires further study as this chapter only presents a descriptive analysis of preliminary findings and selected responses to individual questions.

Materials and Methods

A clinical examination was completed on 607 15–17-year-old males and females. They also completed a questionnaire. Two returns were unsatisfactory in relation to social stratification.

Table 8.1   Social Class Position Matrix (*McGreil*[9]).

	1 Post- grad. (4)	2 Grad. (8)	3 In- complete U/grad. (12)	4 Complete second (16)	5 In- complete second (20)	6 Complete primary (24)	7 In- complete primary (28)
1. High professional etc. (7)	I 11	I 15	II 19	II 23	II 27	II 31	III 35
2. Executive, etc. (14)	II 18	II 22	II 26	II 30	III 34	III 38	III 42
3. High inspect., etc. (21)	II 25	II 29	III 33	III 37	III 41	III 45	IV 49
4. Supervisory, etc. (28)	III 32	III 36	III 40	III 44	IV 48	IV 52	IV 56
5. Skilled-man., routine non-manual (35)	III 39	III 43	III 47	IV 51	IV 55	IV 59	IV 63
6. Semi-skilled manual (42)	III 46	IV 50	IV 54	IV 58	IV 62	V 66	V 70
7. Unskilled manual (49)	IV 53	IV 57	IV 61	V 65	V 69	V 73	V 77

Selection of subjects

A list of all secondary schools in Dublin was divided into five groups based on a preliminary assessment of social stratification. Schools were then randomly selected from each one of the five groups to provide a sample of males and females. Participants completed a questionnaire and were given a form to bring to their parents for completion to provide the required information on their parents' education and employment, together with consent for their child undergoing a clinical examination. There was a bias in this method towards compliance, since approval had to be sought for the examination.

Socio-Educational Matrix (SEM)

The subjects' socio-educational position was based on the occupation and education of the parent providing the main source of income in the household. The combination of education and occupation is the most reliable criterion of social class position in modern society.[9] *Hollingshead*[6] classified education and occupation on two 7-point ordinal scales. He weighted education by 4 and occupation by 7 and combined the scores to provide a potential numerical range between 11 and 77. He then divided the scores into a 5-interval 'social position scale'. *McGreil* in his work on *Prejudice and Tolerance in Ireland*[9] modified this matrix for a survey in Dublin and that modification was the basis for designating social class position in this study (Table 8.1).

Clinical examination

Two examiners participated in the examination. One scored the DMFT and the second completed a periodontal examination which included a plaque score, a gingival bleeding index and pocket measurements. The examiners standardized scoring prior to the study. The DMFT was scored using the criteria laid down by WHO in 1977.[18]

In the periodontal examination the third molar teeth were excluded. Plaque was scored as follows:

0 no detectable plaque
1 plaque detectable with probe only (mild)
2 visible plaque deposits (visible)

Gingival bleeding was scored by drawing a periodontal probe with a 0.5 mm diameter tip[17] along the gingival crevice from the mesiolingual aspect of each tooth distally and from the distobuccal aspect mesially, finally recording the pocket depth interproximally from the mesiobuccal aspect. This was done on a quadrant basis and bleeding was recorded as being present on the lingual, buccal, or both lingual and buccal aspect of each tooth.

Pocket depth

Pocket depth was recorded interproximally from the mesiobuccal aspect of each tooth[17] as follows:

0 < 4 mm
1 4– 5 mm
2 > 6 mm.

Questionnaire

Preliminary studies were undertaken to develop a questionnaire. This was divided into groups of questions related to the following:

1. Dental health principles
2. Stated attitudes
3. Stated behaviour in relation to:
   (a) professional care
   (b) oral hygiene practices
   (c) diet
4. Perception of dental health status.

The questionnaire will be the subject of a more detailed analysis, but it was thought appropriate to report the responses to some individual questions at this workshop.

Results

Socio-Educational Matrix (SEM)

In Table 8.2 the group is divided into five socio-educational (SEM) groups. *McGreil's* random sample of Dublin adults[9] is also included for the purpose of comparison. Our study had more subjects in the higher SEM groups than reported in *McGreil's* random sample. This was anticipated in view of the sampling method used and the fact that all were attending secondary school. There was a disproportionate total number of males (63.3%) to females (36.7%) and also a significantly higher proportion of females in the SEM groups I and II.

Gingival bleeding

The intraoral distribution of stimulated gingival bleeding is presented in Fig. 8.1. This also illustrates bleeding free units and demonstrates that there is relatively little bleeding from first premolar to first premolar. The buccal aspect of mandibular teeth is relatively free from gingival bleeding. It is interesting to note the prevalence of gingival bleeding lingual to the mandibular premolar and molar teeth and also on the buccal and palatal aspect of the maxillary

111

Table 8.2 Distribution of SEM groups in this study compared to the random sample of Dublin adults (McGreil[9]).

| | Present study, (15–17-year-olds) | | | | McGreil's adult sample |
	All %	Males %	Females %	Number	All %
Group I	16	9	8	99	3
Group II	16	9	7	95	11
Group III	20	15	6	124	19
Group IV	37	25	12	224	46
Group V	10	7	4	63	21
Total	99	63	37	605	100%

Table 8.3 Frequency distribution of the percentage of bleeding sites following probing in the entire sample. Bleeding was scored on buccal and lingual aspects of each tooth.

Distribution of sample with bleeding %	Bleeding sites %
28	0
29	1–10
21	11–20
15	21–40
7	41% or more

Table 8.4 Comparison of bleeding between the five SEM groups and between males and females.

	Mean %	s.d.[1]
Group I	9.4	13.7
Group II	10.8	15.0
Group III	13.0	16.0
Group IV	14.9	17.2
Group V	12.4	14.3
Males	14.7	16.5
Females	9.3	14.3
Entire Population	12.8	16.0

[1] s.d. = standard deviation

second premolar and molar teeth. The distribution of bleeding makes an interesting comparison with Fig. 8.2 (plaque) and Fig. 8.3 (pocketing). Table 8.3 shows a frequency distribution of the percentage of bleeding sites in the sample.

Bleeding and SEM

The mean bleeding score for the five SEM groups and also the mean bleeding index for males and females is presented in Table 8.4. By dividing the sample into four groups of zero, low, medium and high bleeding, an association was found between bleeding and SEM grouping (Table 8.5). Those in the lower SEM groups had more bleeding than those in the higher ones. However, this difference was not found in males but was shown to be related in females (Table 8.6). In other words, female gingival bleeding was associated with SEM grouping, while male gingival bleeding was not. Table 8.7 shows the analysis of SEM by the sexes.

Plaque

The distribution of plaque is illustrated in Fig. 8.2. This demonstrates a greater ac-

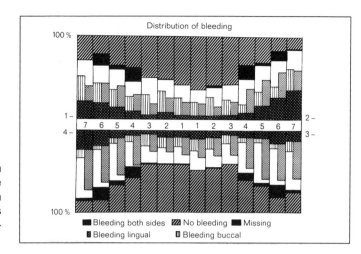

Fig. 8.1 Intraoral distribution of bleeding and bleeding-free sites following probing with WHO 621 probe in 607 males and females (15–17-year-olds).

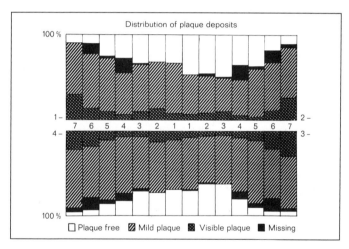

Fig. 8.2 Intraoral distribution of plaque deposits 607 males and females (15–17-year-olds).

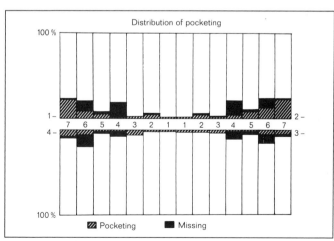

Fig. 8.3 Distribution of periodontal pocketing (4–5 mm) in 607 males and females (15–17-year-olds).

Table 8.5   Bleeding by SEM groupings – male and female combined.

| | | | SEM Groupings | | | |
Bleeding	I	II	III	IV	V	Total
0	34	34	37	45	20	170
Low	36	20	36	69	12	173
Medium	16	29	21	50	15	131
High	13	12	30	60	16	131
Total	99	95	124	224	63	605

χ^2 (d.f. = 12) = 31.98. **P** < 0.01

Table 8.6   Bleeding by SEM groupings – females.

| | | | SEM Groupings | | | |
Bleeding	I	II	III	IV	V	Total
0	22	24	14	17	9	86
Low	18	10	12	25	5	70
Medium	4	7	4	16	4	35
High	3	2	5	17	5	32
Total	47	43	35	75	23	223

χ^2 (d.f. = 12) = 24.50. **P** < 0.01

Table 8.7   Bleeding by male and female.

Bleeding	Male	Female	Total
0	85	86	171
Low	103	70	173
Medium	96	35	131
High	100	32	132
Total	384	223	607

χ^2 (d.f. = 3) = 29.08. **P** < 0.001

cumulation on the right side, but otherwise a distribution similar to Fig. 8.2. Table 8.8 shows the frequency distribution of the percentage of teeth with plaque deposits. Eighty-four per cent of the group had plaque deposits on more than half of the number of teeth in their mouth and 18% had plaque on all of their teeth. On average, 21 out of the 28 teeth per mouth examined had plaque deposits.

Table 8.8 Frequency distribution of teeth with plaque deposits for the entire sample.

Teeth with plaque %	% of sample
100	18
90– 99	15
80– 89	15
70– 79	15
60– 69	10
50– 59	11
30– 50	10
< 30	6

Table 8.9 Comparison of mean plaque deposition in the five SEM groups and in males and females.

	Mean %	s.d.[1]
Group I	67.7	23.8
Group II	70.0	26.8
Group III	72.3	24.6
Group IV	77.1	21.7
Group V	78.2	19.1
Males	78.3	21.8
Females	65.3	24.3
Entire Population	73.6	23.5

[1] s.d. = standard deviation

Table 8.10 Distribution of plaque deposition by SEM.

	SEM Groupings					
Plaque	I	II	III	IV	V	Total
Low	14	16	17	18	3	68
Medium	22	16	23	29	7	97
High	47	42	54	112	38	293
Maximum	16	21	30	65	15	147
Total	99	95	124	224	63	605

χ^2 (d.f. = 12) = 21.52. **P** < 0.05

Plaque and SEM

Table 8.9 shows the mean plaque score for the five SEM groups and also for males and females. Males have a higher score for plaque than females. There was evidence that plaque deposition was heavier in the lower SEM groups (Table 8.10). Males were shown to have a significantly higher percentage of teeth with plaque deposition than females (Table 8.11).

Table 8.11 Distribution of plaque deposits by males and females.

Plaque	Male	Female	Total
Low	29	40	69
Medium	55	42	97
High	178	116	294
Maximum	122	25	147
Total	384	223	607

χ^2 (d.f. = 3) = 40.74. **P** < 0.001

115

Table 8.12 % of subjects with pocketing 4 mm – 5 mm.

% of sample	Number of pockets
48	0
20	1
12	2
10	3
8	4

Pocketing

The oral distribution of pocketing is illustrated in Fig. 8.3 and Table 8.12 presents the frequency distribution of pocketing in the sample. Pockets were scored interproximally from the mesiobuccal aspect of each tooth and the pattern of distribution of pocketing reflects the distribution of bleeding (Fig. 8.1) and plaque deposition (Fig. 8.2). In comparing the results of bleeding and pocketing one should refer to the bar graph, which represents bleeding on the buccal aspect of the teeth, because pocket depths were only recorded on the buccal aspect. Only four pockets of 6 mms or more were recorded in the entire population. Forty-eight per cent of individuals had no pockets deeper than 4 mm.

Pocketing and SEM

While females were shown to have a lower incidence of pocketing than males, there was no difference seen in the incidence of pocketing between the five SEM groups.

DMFT

Table 8.13 presents a summary of the findings and shows the very low mean DMFT consistent with other studies in Ireland.[4] This will be the subject of a paper by *Frances Ahern* (the second author, of this review), but it is of interest to note that no association was found between SEM and DMFT. Females were found to have a higher DMF than males although a lower D/DMF than males. Those in the higher SEM groups had lower D/DMF ratios also. There was a positive correlation between F/DMF and SEM.

Questionnaire

The following questions have been abstracted from the questionnaire and presented as individual responses. This gives some insight to respondents stated attitudes and behaviour.

Table 8.13 Comparison of mean DMFT, D/DMF and F/DMF between SEM groups and between males and females.

	DMFT Mean	s.d.	D/DMF Mean	s.d.	F/DMF Mean	s.d.[1]
Entire Population	5.06	3.5	17.2	28.4	63.6	39.7
Group I	5.23	3.4	11.5	24.7	78.1	34.9
Group II	5.21	3.4	10.9	20.6	71.3	37.5
Group III	4.63	3.5	19.3	31.7	62.0	39.9
Group IV	5.18	3.5	19.6	29.6	59.6	39.7
Group V	5.02	3.7	23.1	30.6	46.1	40.9
Males	4.8	3.4	18.9	29.3	61.9	39.7
Females	5.5	3.6	14.4	26.7	66.3	37.7

[1] s.d. = standard deviation

Q 24. Gum disease cannot be treated.

True	15%
Don't know	43%
False	43%

Q 25. Healthy gums should not bleed after brushing.

True	57%
Don't know	18%
False	25%

Q 28. While sweets are bad for teeth, it is not fair to deprive children of such a pleasure.

Strongly agree	13%
Agree	46%
Not sure	10%
Disagree	23%
Strongly Disagree	8%

Q 36. The quality of life must be less when you lose your teeth.

Strongly agree	12%
Agree	25%
Not sure	16%
Disagree	28%
Strongly disagree	20%

Q 40. How often do you brush your teeth?

a) Rarely, or never	3%
b) Once weekly	4%
c) About every second day	10%
d) Once a day	33%
e) Twice a day or more	49%

Q 49. When did you last visit a dentist for treatment?

a) Never been	3%
b) More than 2 years ago	29%
c) Between 1–2 years	14%
d) Less than 1 year ago	19%
e) Less than 6 months ago	16%
f) Less than 3 months ago	22%

Q 53. Do you believe that you have holes in your teeth (decay)?

a) Certain	19%
b) I think so	19%
c) Don't know	18%
d) Don't think so	27%
e) Certain I don't	18%

Q 54. Do you believe that you have gum disease?

a) Certain	1%
b) I think so	4%
c) Don't know	25%
d) Don't think so	39%
e) Certain I don't	32%

Q 56. Are you making a good enough effort to care for your teeth?

a) Certain	15%
b) I think so	45%
c) Don't know	12%
d) Don't think so	23%
e) Certain I don't	4%

Q 58. Do your gums bleed when you brush your teeth?

a) Never	38%
b) Sometimes	55%
c) Almost always	6%
d) Never brush	1%

While a preliminary analysis of responses to the questionnaire has been completed in relation to SEM grouping it was not thought appropriate to include it in this paper and further analysis will be required before drawing any conclusions.

Discussion

It would be premature to draw firm conclusions on the inter-relationships between the clinical findings, the socio-education groupings and responses to the questionnaire. This will require a more sophisticated factor analysis of the data from the questionnaire. However, the results provide basic information on the pattern of dental disease affecting this age group.

The intraoral distribution of gingival bleeding in Fig. 8.1 is similar to the distribution of plaque (Fig. 8.2) and to a lesser extent to pocketing (Fig. 8.3) found in the sample. This population had more bleeding in two specific areas:

1. The lingual aspect of mandibular teeth.
2. Maxillary first and second molar teeth.

The difference between buccal and lingual bleeding on the mandibular arch was striking. Also, there was less bleeding on the buccal aspect of the left side compared to the buccal aspect of the right side. This was thought to be related to more effective brushing on the left side. There was little bleeding on anterior teeth and on the buccal aspect of all the mandibular teeth.

The intraoral distribution of attachment loss in adults has been reported as being marked in the mandibular anterior teeth[19] unlike the pattern of pocketing and bleeding in this sample. It is possible that the retention of mandibular teeth in adults, together with the cumulative effects of peri-odontal disease, might be responsible for the differences noted compared to this adolescent group. At this stage, despite the time of eruption, the mandibular teeth are among the least affected teeth by gingival bleeding and pocketing.

The differences noted between bleeding on the two central incisors is accounted for by the way in which bleeding was scored in each quadrant. When the 1–8 was first probed in the right maxillary quadrant, the remaining seven teeth had to be probed before returning to 1–8 to see if it was bleeding. This was done in the reverse direction on the left maxillary quadrant. Hence, the 1–1 and 2–8 had less time to demonstrate bleeding than 1–8 or 2–1.

The results illustrate how dental diseases and dental treatment are mainly found around the first permanent molars, while patient self-care, based on plaque control and bleeding free sites, is confined to the anterior regions. More emphasis might be placed on self-diagnosis and effective plaque control in those areas in which higher bleeding scores were recorded in primary preventive programmes in this particular age group.

Despite the prevalence of bleeding and the relatively low DMFT, only 5% of the respondents to the questionnaire thought they had 'gum disease', while 38% thought they had dental caries. It seemed that in this population, subjects did not have an accurate perception of their own dental health problems. They had a greater awareness of dental caries, but were relatively unaware of gingivitis.

One quarter of the population did not appear to appreciate that healthy gingiva should not bleed following brushing. Eighty-two per cent of the sample claimed they brushed their teeth at least daily or more and 60% of the group believed they were making a good-enough effort to care for their teeth. Despite this, three-quarters of all teeth had plaque deposits.

There are certain trends emerging in relation to SEM groupings. Those in the lower groups were found to have more bleeding, more plaque, more decay, fewer fillings, but similar DMFT scores and pocketing to higher groups. Females accounted for the SEM difference in relation to bleeding and it might be speculated that this finding could be related to the earlier maturation of females and, as a consequence, a greater SEM influence. Unfortunately, the sampling was unevenly divided between males and females in the SEM groups. It is a finding which warrants further analysis. Females emerged as having lower plaque scores, higher DMF, lower bleeding, lower D/DMF than males. Females were also less assertive in responding to questions.

It was interesting to compare respondents' stated intentions with their actual behaviour in relation to professional dental care. While 47% intended to visit a dentist within the next few months, only 22% had visited one within the past 3 months. In relation to social stratification, the lower SEM groups did not visit as regularly as the higher SEM groups, but their intentions were almost as good as those in the higher SEM groups to do so in the future. There is an old Irish saying that 'The road to Hell is paved with good intentions'.

When a factor-analysis has been completed on grouped questions in the questionnaire it will be possible to analyse stated attitudes and behaviour in relation to the social stratification of the subjects and the clinical findings.

report is mainly concerned with the clinical findings.

Periodontal disease and gingival bleeding was scored using the WHO 621 probe. Bleeding was found to be most severe on the lingual aspect of the mandibular molar teeth and on the buccal and palatal aspects of the maxillary second premolar and molar teeth. It is suggested that there should be greater emphasis on self-diagnosis of gingival bleeding in those sites at risk to higher levels of bleeding and patients were advised how to carry out effective hygiene in the particular sites. The intraoral distribution of gingival bleeding and pocketing did not reflect the intraoral distribution of attachment loss reported in adults, particularly in mandibular anterior regions.

Although three quarters of all teeth examined had plaque on them, 82% claimed they brushed their teeth at least daily. Only 5% of the sample thought they had gum disease, despite the high incidence of gingival bleeding, while 38% believed they had dental caries.

Those in the lower socio-educational groups had more plaque, more caries, fewer restorations than those in the higher groups, although no significant difference was found in DMFT scores. Females had higher DMFT scores and lower gingival bleeding scores than males. Social stratification influenced the levels of gingival bleeding significantly in female subjects but not so in males. Females had higher F/DMF than males.

Patients' intentions to pursue treatment or care were not reliable and were overstated.

Summary

A study was carried out on 607 adolescents in Dublin to determine levels of dental health and the influence of socio-educational factors. The study incorporated a detailed questionnaire, but this preliminary report is mainly concerned with the clinical findings.

Acknowledgements

We wish to acknowledge the support of the Medical Research Council of Ireland and the Board of the Dublin Dental Hospital.

We are grateful to Ms *Humphries* and Ms *McColl,* Trinity College, for the statistical analysis. We are indebted to the Dental Nurses and Ms *Merry* for their help in the study and to Drs *Sheiham* and *O'Hickey* for their advice.

References

1. *Ainamo J., Barmes D. E., Beagrie G., Cutress T.* and *Martin J.*
   Development of The World Health Organization (WHO) Community Periodontal Index of Treatment Needs (CPITN). Int. Dent. J., 1982, 32: 281–291.

2. *Anderson R. J., James P. M. C., James, D. M.* and *Norden, H.*
   Dental Caries Experience and Treatment Pattern. Brit. Dent. J., 1971, 131: 67–71.

3. *Bulman J. S., Richards M. D., Stack G. L.* and *Willcock A. J.*
   Demand and Need for Dental Care. Oxford University Press, 1968.

4. *Butler N. P., O'Mullane D.* and *O'Hickey S.*
   Report on the International Collaborative Study in Ireland. Paper presented at Odontological Section of Royal College of Medicine of Ireland, Jan. 1982.

5. *Frandsen A.*
   Educational objectives in relation to the provision of care. In Efficacy of Treatment Procedures in Periodontics. (Shanley D. B., ed.) Quintessence, Berlin, 1980, pp. 251–268.

6. *Hollingshead A. B.* and *Redlick F. C.*
   Social Class and Mental Illness. A Community Study. Wiley & Sons, New York, 1956.

7. *Kiyak H. A.*
   Dental beliefs, behaviour and health status among Pacific Asians and Caucasians. Community Dent. Oral Epidemiol., 1981, 9: 10–14.

8. *Lennon M. A.* and *Davies R. M.*
   Prevalence and distribution of alveolar bone loss in a population of 15 year-old school children. J. Clin. Periodontol., 1974, 1: 175–182.

9. *McGreil M.*
   Prejudice and Tolerance in Ireland. College of Industrial Relation, Dublin, 1977.

10. *Nikias M. K., Fink R.* and *Sollecito W.*
    Oral health status in relation to socio-economic and ethnic characteristics of urban adults in the U.S.A. Community Dent. Oral Epidemiol., 1977, 5: 200–206.

11. *Pilot T.*
    Analysis of the overall effectiveness of treatment of periodontal disease. In Efficacy of Treatment Procedures in Periodontics. (Shanley D. B. ed.) Quintessence, Berlin, 1980, pp. 213–230.

12. *Shanley D. B. (ed.)*
    Efficacy of Treatment Procedures in Periodontics. Quintessence, Berlin, 1980.

13. *Sheiham A.*
    Current Concepts in Health Education. In Efficacy of Treatment Procedures in Periodontics. (Shanley, D. B., ed.) Quintessence, Berlin, 1980, pp. 23–40.

14. *Sheiham A., Maizels J. E.* and *Cushing A. M.*
    1982 The concept of need in dental care. Int. Dent. J., 1982, 32: 265–270.

15. *Sutcliffe P.*
    Caries experience and oral cleanliness of 3- and 4-year-old children from deprived and nondeprived areas in Edinburgh, Scotland. Community Dent. Oral Epidemiol., 1977, 5: 213–219.

16. *Sutherland D. A.* and *Stephens K. W.*
    Relationship between social class and dental health in 14 year-old children. J. Dent. Res., 1971, 50: 1185.

17. *World Health Organization.*
    Epidemiology Etiology and Prevention of Periodontal Diseases. Tech. Rep. Series No. 621, Geneva, 1978.

18. *World Health Organization.*
    Oral Health Surveys, Basic Methods. 2nd ed., Geneva, 1977.

19. *Waerhaug J.*
    Epidemiology of Periodontal Disease. Review of literature. In World Workshop in Periodontics. Ramfjord, S. et al. eds.). Ann Arbor, Michigan, 1966.

9. Goals for Periodontal Health and Acceptable Levels of Disease: Means and Methods in Community Strategies

Per Gjermo

Introduction

Recently, the World Health Organization (WHO) has encouraged the establishment of defined goals within the various fields of health by launching the slogan: *Health for all in the year 2000.* Dental health goals are in the process of being established, in cooperation with the FDI (Fédération Dentaire Internationale). The idea of defining such goals, which should be regarded as guidelines for public health planners and politicians, is attractive. However, whereas the WHO's intention is to describe a global goal valid for the total population of the world, operative goals restricted for subpopulations within countries may be more useful in the Western European industrialized communities.

Periodontal disease is evident in all countries at moderate to high levels and in many populations results in extensive loss of teeth among adults.[18, 36, 47, 53, 55] The early signs of the disease appear during the teenage period, and a prevalence of 10% and more of subjects with bone loss at the age of 15 is not uncommon (Fig. 9.1).[11, 25, 38] On the other hand, recent reports indicate that regular dental care, with the emphasis on prevention, may reduce the disease prevalence and severity.[25, 35, 40] Apparently, the knowledge accumulated during recent years, which has provided a rational explanation of the initiation and progression of chronic marginal periodontitis, seems to be adequate for the control of the disease at the individual and community level.

In order to establish community programmes to prevent and treat periodontitis, it is mandatory to know the disease status in the target population. Based on the actual disease situation, realistic and scientifically sound goals for periodontal health in the future may be agreed upon and strategies developed by which goals can be reached.

Various aspects of periodontal care and periodontal health, including ways of describing periodontal health goals and acceptable levels of disease, are discussed here. Furthermore, means and methods which may be used to develop community strategies are suggested. The discussion is mainly concerned with programmes related to children and young adults who may easily be reached through the school systems in well-organized societies. Systematic dental health care, with emphasis on prevention, should initially be targeted towards these young populations in the hope that this will reduce the long term needs for the treatment of periodontitis.

Periodontal Care

Periodontal care may be separated into three main areas:

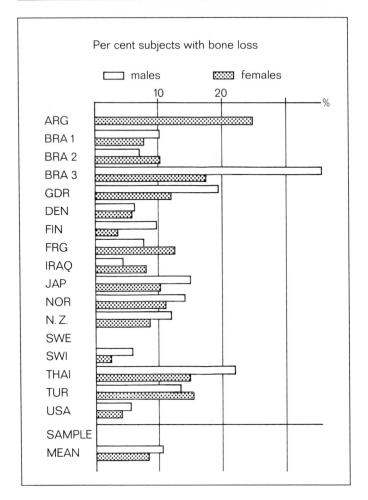

Fig. 9.1 Per cent of 15-year-old subjects from 17 different geographic locations with bone loss on bite-wing roentgenograms (from Hansen et al.[25]).

1. A self-administered oral hygiene regimen, which, in the absence of plaque retentive factors such as calculus and overhanging dental restorations will lead to minimal accumulations of plaque at the gingival margin and the absence of gingival inflammation.[7, 42]

2. Simple treatment procedures performed by dental auxiliary personnel, such as dental hygienists, and involving the removal of plaque retentive factors and the control of subgingival plaque in pockets of moderate depth (3–5 mm). Recurrence of the disease will be prevented by a self-administered oral hygiene regimen.

3. Complex periodontal *treatment* requiring the technical skill and experience of highly trained professionals (dentists) and involving the management of inflamed deep periodontal pockets with advanced loss of supporting tissue. Once restored, the maintenance of periodontal health in most cases will be achieved by self-administered care, and/or by regular professional care by dentists or auxiliaries.[7]

Periodontal condition	CPITN score	Type of care	CPITN TN*	Personnel
Healthy	0	None	0	None
Gingivitis	1	OHE**	1	Teachers/ dental auxiliaries
Calculus	2	OHE + scaling	2	Dental auxiliaries/ dentists
Pockets 3–5 mm	3	OHE + scalling	2	Dental auxiliaries/ dentists
Pockets >5 mm	4	OHE + complex treatment	3	Dentists

* Treatment category
** Oral health education (oral hygiene instruction)

Fig. 9.2 The Community Periodontal Index for Treatment Need (CPITN) as related to type of care and personnel requirements.

Evaluation of Need for Care

Based on the above approaches to periodontal care, the Periodontal Treatment Need System (PTNS) was introduced in 1973.[37] The PTNS may be used for treatment planning in population groups and estimation of time and personnel requirements,[10] provided the average time needed to perform the various treatment procedures is known.[9] Recently, a modification of this system, the Community Periodontal Index for Treatment Need (CPITN), has been developed by a WHO expert group[55] and later by a Joint WHO/ FDI Working Group.[3] A specially designed periodontal probe is recommended for the scoring procedures.[15] The CPITN is based on the examination of six segments (sextants) of the dentition and provides a simple and reliable method for estimation of treatment needs. The collection of data using the CPITN has already started,[22] and in a short time it is hoped that the periodontal treatment needs in many countries will be described according to these criteria. The importance of such data for the planning and implementation of health services cannot be underestimated.[8] Moreover, the CPITN may be used by health authorities to describe periodontal

health goals by describing acceptable levels of need for treatment in subgroups of a population, and to set priorities according to available resources. The relationship between different entities of periodontal care and the CPITN is schematically shown in Fig. 9.2.

Periodontal Care Strategies

Education

The most important part of periodontal care on a population basis is the self-administered oral hygiene. The success of this part of the care is dependent not only on the attitudes and values of the population in question,[12, 45] but also on its factual knowledge. In the Scandinavian countries, information of dental health is given to parents of small children and directly to primary school children as part of their school programme.[30, 33] However, there are indications that children's and adults' knowledge of caries is much better than their knowledge of gingivitis and periodontitis.[1, 44, 49] As a first step, goals for the knowledge of oral health that should be gained during primary school should be defined in cooperation with the responsible authorities. Systematic use of mass media will increase the background knowledge and alertness of the population and the profession. In Norway, the Dental Association initiated a 'perio-year' in 1981 on a nationwide scale.[46] During the first half of the year, emphasis was given to postgraduate courses and information to the profession. Approximately 50% of all Norwegian dentists took part in such courses.[51] In the second half of the year, the target group was the total population and a professional press agency was involved to carry the messages through all types of mass media.[50]

Gingivitis

It is generally accepted that although gingivitis is a prerequisite for the initiation of a destructive periodontitis, it does not always lead to loss of periodontal attachment. In spite of some recent data indicating an association between the degree of gingivial inflammation and bone loss in young adults,[5] no methods are at present available to distinguish the 'dangerous' gingivitis from the 'innocent' one.

However, gingivitis is a result of accumulation of bacterial plaque along the gingival margin and therefore the prevalence and spread of gingivitis in the dentition reflect the level of oral hygiene in the individual, as well as on a population level.

In many industrialized countries, the importance of toothbrushing has been emphasized for many years with a certain success, whereas interdental cleaning has been more or less neglected. In such populations, papillitis may be a useful indicator of oral hygiene.

Poor oral hygiene can hardly be regarded as a disease, but it constitutes a threat against dental health and may lead to bad breath[54] and bleeding gums.[41, 42] Such conditions per se are not acceptable in a modern society, and their reduction

should be an integrated part of oral health care programmes.[24] However, both the systematic selection of those with a high need for oral hygiene improvements and evaluation of programmes have been hampered by the lack of suitable index systems. Existing indices for plaque and gingivitis are constructed mainly for experimental or epidemiological purposes[29, 43] and therefore not well suited for application in regular public dental health care programmes.

Recently, a simplified system, the Non-Bleeding Papillae (NBP)[13, 28] has been introduced as part of the public dental care programme for 14–16-year-olds in a community outside Oslo.[24] According to the NBP-system, gingivitis is recorded when bleeding from the papilla occurs after the insertion of a wooden toothpick interdentally (Fig. 9.3). The degree of gingival health and oral hygiene is then recorded as percentages of NBP. In spite of the lack of information of the gingival condition on the lingual and vestibular surfaces by this method, a pilot study indicated that, on a group basis, NBP provided the same information of the gingival health as a complete Gingival Index (GI), according to Löe,[39] or a modification based on a dicotomization of the GI.[4] On an individual basis, the NBP revealed a somewhat smaller difference between those with a very high and a very low GI.[24] This may be explained by papillitis also being prevalent among dedicated toothbrushers. The importance of emphasizing interdental cleaning is thus supported.

When applied in our test community it was revealed that the majority of our target group displayed between 30% and 60% NBP (Fig. 9.4). However, some students showed less than 30% NBP and we decided arbitrarily that this indicated an unacceptable level of oral hygiene. These subjects were then selected and, on a group basis, given oral health education (OHE) with emphasis on interdental cleaning by dental hygienists.[6] The result was

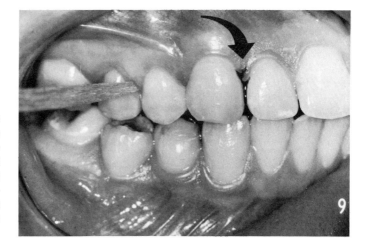

Fig. 9.3 Scoring procedure for the Non-Bleeding Papillae (NBP) system. Bleeding (arrow) occurs after withdrawal of the tooth pick. Papillae which do not bleed after provocation with a wooden toothpick are regarded as healthy (from Gjermo & Moe[24]).

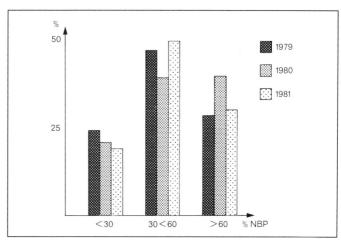

Fig. 9.4 Distribution of schoolchildren aged 14–16 years according to per cent Non-Bleeding Papillae (NBP) over 3 years (from Gjermo & Moe[24]).

an immediate improvement of approximately 40% NBP (Table 9.1) and after one year only 17% of the subjects initially included in the programme were again selected for the OHE programme (Table 9.2).[24]

During the 3 years this system has been implemented, a total of 135 students have been selected for the OHE programme. All of them have accepted the offer and cooperated well. The total cost of the programme for these 3 years can be estimated as approximately 37 dental hygienist hours.[24]

Both the dentists performing the annual routine examination, which was the basis for selection, and the dental hygienists who carried out the OHE programme, found the NBP-system easy and simple to use. Furthermore, they reported that the provoked bleeding *per se* had a motivating and explanatory effect upon the participants. The reduced bleeding from the papillae, which could be shown and quantified after a short time of implementation of interdental cleaning procedures, was appreciated as a reward by students as well as by dentists and hygienists.

Table 9.1 Non-Bleeding Papillae (NBP) before and after group therapy by dental hygienists in 14 – 16-year-old children with a poor oral hygiene (from Gjermo & Moe[24]).

Year	Age	N	Mean NBP before %	after %	Increase in NBP %
1979	16	45	14.1	47.1	33.0
1980	15	65	18.6	63.8	45.2
1981	14	25	14.5	56.2	41.7
Total	14 – 16	135	16.3	56.8	40.5

Thus, both parts were encouraged to further efforts. To use gingival bleeding to visualize gingivitis, and motivate improved oral hygiene, has been recommended by several authors.[2, 4, 31]

The proposed NBP system seems suited for systematized selection of children with a particular need for improved interdental hygiene. The percentage of NBP may also be easily monitored longitudinally in order to evaluate programmes in individual subjects, as well as in groups and populations. It is also evident that the NBP system can be used for assessing the acceptable level of disease (gingivitis) and oral hygiene in populations according to present status, available resources and priorities, thus forming the basis of sub-

Table 9.2 Longterm effect of 4 weeks (4 sessions) of group therapy by dental hygienists on the prevalence of Non-Bleeding Papillae (NBP) among 15-year-old schoolchildren with initial poor oral hygiene and the number of children with unacceptable oral hygiene (<30% NBP) (from Gjermo & Moe[24]).

	Before	After 6 weeks	After 1 Year
Hean NBP (%)	18.6	63.8	49.4
No of children w/ <30% NBP	65	1	11

goals for periodontal health. The demand for such data is high, since they are virtually nonexistent even in the Scandinavian countries where systematic dental care programmes for school children have been in action for more than 50 years. [16]

Periodontitis

Primary prevention of periodontitis would imply complete control of gingivitis but, with the present methods, this is regarded impractical, if not impossible, on a population basis.[19] Consequently, a certain level of gingivitis might be accepted. An example of how such levels may be described is given above.

It has been recommended that secondary prevention, i.e. early diagnosis, treatment of incipient disease and prevention of recurrence in susceptible individuals, should be the principle of choice in public dental care for periodontal disease.[19, 20] The early detection of destructive disease increases the possibilities of successful management. The procedures involved can be administered by auxiliary personnel and is less time-consuming and expensive than the treatment of advanced disease[22] (Fig. 9.2).

Clinical criteria are not suitable to identify individuals with destructive disease in young populations.[5, 14, 22, 26, 32] In an international survey it has been shown that

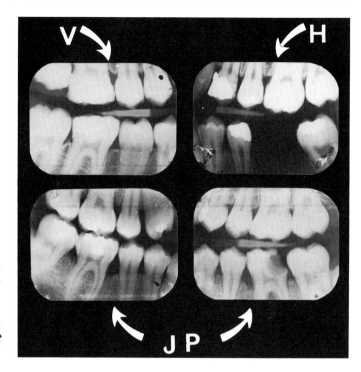

Fig. 9.5 Examples of bite-wing roentgenograms with incipient bone loss. V = vertical lesion, H = horizontal lesion, JP = juvenile periodontitis type lesion (from Gjermo *et al.*[23]).

10–15% of 15-year-olds display bone loss on radiographs[11, 25] (Fig. 9.1). It has been suggested that those with radiographic bone loss at this early age should be regarded as subjects at risk and be given priority for care.[19, 20, 22, 23, 34, 38] It is therefore recommended that screening of young populations should include radiographic assessments, and bite-wing roentgenograms seem suitable for that purpose (Fig. 9.5).[14, 20, 21, 22, 26, 38, 48] The resources necessary to deliver adequate care may be calculated by employing the CPITN with the modifications suggested by *Gjermo et al.*[22] and priority given to those with bone loss.

Advanced periodontal disease is rare in young adults, and the prevalence of juvenile periodontitis is probably close to 0.1%.[25, 48] From a public health planner's point of view, this disease entity is not important as far as time consumption and resource requirements are concerned, but constitutes a challenge to the screening methods for early diagnosis. Since this disease usually involves the first molars, bitewing radiographs are probably very useful for this purpose (Fig. 9.5).

In a longitudinal study employing bitewing roentgenograms, less than 50% of the subjects displaying bone lesions at the age of 15 showed an increase in number of lesions 6 years later (Table 9.3) and in no case had severe changes of existing lesions taken place during this time. These findings indicate that a systematic longitudinal approach of employing radiographs may further limit the number of subjects with a high need for care and thus be valuable for the setting of priorities and allocation of resources. Thus, regular x-ray screening, in combination with the use of the CPITN for estimation of the amount of care needed, seems to be the

Table 9.3 Subjects with and without increased number of sites with bone loss on bitewing roentgenograms from 1975 to 1981 (N = 550, age in 1975 = 15 years).

	Number of subjects	%
Increase	16	42.1
No increase	22	57.9

choice in periodontal care for age groups above 20 years of age. At older ages (35 and over), priority of care should be given to those scoring 4 according to the CPITN (Fig. 9.2) since this may constitute a risk of losing teeth due to periodontal destruction.

Implementation of periodontal care on a community level

In order to apply a systematic dental care programme to a population, or to target groups within a population, it is necessary to establish a well-functioning organization. In many developed countries, some kind of school dental service, or military dental service, has been organized to meet this demand.

The first organized community programme for school children was implemented in Oslo early this century.[30] Since then a rapid development of this kind of service has taken place in the Scandinavian countries and, at present, they are probably among the leading countries in the field of systematic dental care for children and young adults.[17] In the early phase of this development, the services rendered were mainly aiming at pain relief. Later on, as caries became an increasing problem, restorative care dominated. Due to a high number of well qualified dentists, a well organized dental care delivery system, with clinics in almost all schools and wealthy communities, it was possible to prevent tooth loss to a great extent in young Scandinavians, in spite of having one of the highest caries incidences in the world. However, this way of coping with the caries problem was very expensive and not satisfactory from a dental health point of view. Even if most teeth were present at the age of 20, the DMF was extremely high, and all the fillings created a great need for further restorative services later in life. During the 1960s, it became evident that fillings and restorations *per se* did not reduce the disease activity (i.e. caries incidence). Gingival and periodontal problems had so far been given little or no attention.[16]

By a gradual change in the concept of the management of caries from a predominantly restorative to a preventive one, among the dentists as well as among politicians and the population at large, a dramatic change has taken place in Scandinavia concerning caries prevalence and incidence among children during the 1970s.[16] For various reasons, water fluoridation has been introduced to a very limited extent in the Scandinavian countries. The achievement that have been reached concerning caries have therefore been made possible only through a well organized dental care delivery system, including programmes for topical use of fluorides covering almost 100% of the target population, OHE, and dietary advice.[27, 33]

In societies with a high incidence of caries in children, caries prevention must have a high priority in order to prevent early tooth loss.[21] However, there are indications that periodontal disease is the main cause of tooth loss after the fourth decade of life,[18, 36] and that early destructive periodontitis is common in teenagers.[11] Thus, the results of an effective anti-caries programme may be undermined during adulthood, if due attention is not paid to gingival diseases. Even in the Scandinavian countries, with their well organized public dental health systems, preventive action and systematic programmes aiming at the control of periodontal diseases are scarce and systematic data collection to describe the disease status is lacking.[16] One of the reasons may be the lack of suitable index systems, as mentioned above, but recent reports indicate that these difficulties may be overcome and that good results may be obtained within the existing system.[24, 35] A major task in the near future would therefore naturally be to include systematic prevention and therapeutic periodontal care in the delivery system.

Development of strategies

For a public health planner the ideal way of developing a strategy would be to describe a measureable health goal for the population, which, given unlimited resources, is obtainable from a professional and scientific point of view. Then the necessary requirements for personnel, administration, organization, physical facilities, etc., could be calculated.

Unfortunately, the real situation is usually different. The available resources are clearly finite and nowadays rather limited. The public health planner's task under these circumstances will be to develop a strategy to achieve the highest possible health goal within existing or attainable levels of personnel and organization. Again this will call for a description of subgoals for various subsets of the population. One main tool would be data on current disease status described by suitable treatment need indices. Such data are almost nonexistent, and the first important step would be to collect this kind of information. The CPITN[3] seems to be a suitable instrument for periodontal disease in this respect, with some reservations applicable to young populations.[5, 22] By including bite-wing radiographs as a means of selecting individuals at risk, one study of young adults demonstrated a considerable reduction in need for treatment according to the CPITN.[22]

Goals may be described for certain levels of knowledge about gingival diseases and oral hygiene to be obtained by the population at different ages. The means may be the educational system (schools), media, and the professional team. Evaluation of results may be obtained through tests at school, or by quizzing.

In modern societies it seems acceptable to assess goals for oral hygiene. Poor oral hygiene may not be regarded as a disease, but may enhance the risk for developing oral diseases and also cause subjective discomfort as bleeding gums and bad breath.[41, 42, 54] Since the degree and extent of gingivitis reflect the oral hygiene level of the individual, measurements of the extension of gingivitis may be used for evaluation of efforts to obtain oral hygiene goals. Thus, goals concerning gingivitis may be obtained and described concomitantly with the goals for oral hygiene.

When describing goals for the control of gingivitis in the population, the question of acceptable levels of disease will have to be discussed. For an individual this may be described, for instance, as 'the degree and extent of gingivitis which give no discomfort and do not lead to progressive disease'. However, at present, there is no available methods to discern the gingivitis that will develop into destructive periodontitis from that which will not.[5, 14, 26] Also, this acceptable level of disease may be very difficult to measure at a population level. Therefore, it is recommended to describe the level of acceptable gingivitis (reflecting the oral hygiene) according to available resources.[24]

Periodontitis is common in the second decade of life.[11, 38] However, the treatment of incipient disease is simple and may even be performed by auxiliary personnel. A goal for young population groups (below 20 years of age) might therefore be to diagnose and treat all periodontal disease at an incipient stage, and to regard those individuals showing actual loss of tooth supporting tissue early in life as risk sub-

Table 9.4 Subjects with bone loss on bite-wing roentgenograms in 1975 and 1981 (age in 1975 = 15 years).

Sex	Number	Subjects with bone loss (%)	
		1975	1981
Males	244	19 (7.9)	58 (23.8)
Females	306	19 (6.3)	62 (20.1)
Both	550	38 (6.9)	120 (21.8)

jects with a high priority for care.[19, 20, 22, 23, 34, 38] There are indications that 10–15% of teenagers may be expected to belong to such risk groups[11, 25] and that this figure may be three times higher in the early 20s (Table 9.4).

Goals for periodontal health in older age groups (over 20) may in different ways be described as acceptable levels of need for treatment for instance according to the CPITN[4] (Fig. 9.2). The CPITN data may easily be transcribed into time units needed to provide care[10, 22, 55] or the goals may be described as allowing a certain proportion of subjects or sextants in the defined treatment categories (Fig. 9.2).

When establishing priorities for periodontal care in an adult population, the rate of progression of the disease should be taken into consideration and not only the disease status. At present, no reliable methods for such assessments are available, but periodic assessments of radiographic bone levels may be useful in the clinic. In the future methods for monitoring changes in the flora, for instance, by immunologic techniques[52] may facilitate the selection of subjects needing care.

Acceptable levels of disease

In order to set periodontal health goals for a total population (all ages), certain levels of disease must at present be accepted. A superior goal would be that periodontal disease should not limit the social function (in its widest sense) of the dentition throughout life.

Because in many populations dental function is already reduced by periodontitis, such a description could only be made valid for those who are very young or those who until now have suffered minimal tooth loss or loss of supporting tissues. A difficult problem would be to define the levels of disease at various ages that would be compatible with acceptable social function.

Suggestions

A degree of gingivitis which does not cause spontaneous bleeding or pain could be accepted as a 'normal' reaction against noxious bacterial products.

An extension of gingivitis which does not involve the front region (cosmetic reasons), or cause foetor ex ore at a socially unacceptable level, might also be allowed. This would correspond to CPITN score 0 in the frontal sextants, and a maximum of score 2 in the posterior sextants.

Radiographic bone loss should not be accepted in more than 4 sites, and not represent more than 2 mm loss of attachment at each site in young adults (under 20 years of age). This would imply regular x-ray screening through the teens and is compatible with the finding that more than 3 sites rarely are involved at the age of 15 years[14, 23, 34]

In adults, deep pockets, which according to the CPITN needs dentist expert treatment, should not be accepted. This would mean that subjects showing CPITN score 4 in any sextant should immediately receive proper care. Molars should probably be excluded from evaluation, particularly in subjects over 50 years of age, since no predictable treatment is available when the furcation area of these teeth are severely involved. This may be the case even when the CPITN does not give score 4.

The above acceptable levels of disease should be compatible with a life-long functioning dentition with a minimum use of resources. Most of the efforts will be self-administrated by the patients and most of the professional intervention may be administered by auxiliaries. Dentists should be needed only to a limited degree. However, organized and regular screening of the population is mandatory to achieve any goals on a community level. The first step would be to build up a functioning organization for the delivery of dental health services.

References

1. *Ainamo J.*
   Awareness of the presence of dental caries and gingival inflammation in young adult males. Acta Odontol. Scand., 1972, 30: 615–619.

2. *Ainamo J.*
   The Significance of Periodontal Disease in Society. In Efficacy of Treatment Procedures in Periodontics. (Shanley D. ed.) Quintessence, Berlin, 1980, pp 299–312.

3. *Ainamo J., Barmes D. E., Beagrie G., Cutress T., Martin J.* and *Sardo-Infirri J.*
   Development of the World Health Organization (WHO) Community Periodontal Index of Treatment Needs (CPITN). Int. Dent. J., 1982, 32: 281–291.

4. *Ainamo, J.* and *Bay, I.*
   Problems and proposals for recording gingivitis and plaque. Int. Dent. J. 1975, 25: 229–235.

5. *Albandar J.* and *Gjermo P.*
   Associations between gingivitis, pocket depths and radiographic bone loss in interproximal areas in young adults. Scand. J. Dent. Res., 1983, 91: 371–375.

6. *Arnesen L. B.* and *Simonsen U.*
   Bruk av gingivitt-index (blødnings-index) for utvelgelse av risikopasienter i ungdomsskolen. Effekt av systematisk instruksjon/motivasjon i grupper. Tannstikka, 1981, 7: no 5,7–11.

7. *Axelsson P.* and *Lindhe J.*
   Effect of controlled oral hygiene procedures on caries and periodontal disease in adults. J. Clin. Periodontol. 1978, 5: 133–151.

8. *Barmes D. E.*
   What a public health planner wants from a periodontal assessment. Int. Dent. J., 1976, 26: 429–439.

9. *Bellini H. T.*
   The time factor in periodontal therapy. J. Periodontal Res., 1974, 9: 56–61.

10. *Bellini H. T.* and *Gjermo P.*
    Application of the periodontal treatment need system (PTNS) in a group of Norwegian industrial employees. Community Dent. Oral Epidemiol., 1974, 1: 22–29.

11. *Bellini H. T., Gjermo P.* and *Hansen B. F.*
    International comparative study on the prevalence of bone loss in 15-year-old children. AADR Annual Meeting, 1980, Los Angeles. Abstract no. 121.

12. *Bustad P.*
    Communication and the Prevention of Dental Diseases. In Preventive Dentistry in Practice. (Frandsen A. ed.) Munksgaard, Copenhagen, 1976, pp 114–141.

13. *Dolles O. K.* and *Gjermo P.*
    Caries increment and gingival status during 2 years' use of chlorhexidine- and fluoride-containing dentifrices. Scand. J. Dent. Res., 1980, 88: 22–27.

14. *Ellegaard B.* and *Andersen S. A.*
    En røntgenologisk og klinisk undersøgelse af parodontalt fæstetab omkring 1. molar hos 15-årige. Tandlægebladet, 1979, 83: 115–118.

15. *Emslie R. D.*
    The 621 periodontal probe. Int. Dent. J., 1980, 30: 287–288.

16. *Fehr F. R. v. d.*
    Dental disease in Scandinavia. In Dental Health Care in Scandinavia. (Frandsen A. ed.) Quintessence, Berlin, 1982, pp 21–43.

17. *Frandsen A.*
Dental Health Care in Scandinavia. Quintessence, Berlin, 1982, 5–259.

18. *Gad T.* and *Bay I.*
Årsager til ekstraktion af permanente tænder i Danmark. Tandlægebladet, 1972, 76: 103–114.

19. *Gjermo P.*
Establishment of priorities in periodontal care. In The Efficacy of Treatment Procedures in Periodontics. (Shanley, D. ed.) Quintessence, Berlin, 1980, pp 317–324.

20. *Gjermo P.*
The treatment of periodontal disease in the mixed dentition. Int. Dent. J., 1981, 31: 45–48.

21. *Gjermo P., Beldi M-I., Bellini H. T.* and *Martins C. R.*
Study of tooth loss in an adolescent Brazilian population. Community Dent. Oral Epidemiol., 1983, 11: 371–374.

22. *Gjermo P., Bellini H. T.* and *Marcos B.*
Application of the Community Periodontal Index for Treatment Need (CPITN) in a population of young Brazilians. Community Dent. Oral Epidemiol. 1983, 11: 342–346.

23. *Gjermo P., Bellini H. T., Santos V. P., Martins I. G.* and *Ferracyoli J. R.*
Prevalence of bone loss in a group of Brazilian teenagers assessed on bite-wing radiographs. J. Clin. Periodontol., 1984, 11: 104–113.

24. *Gjermo P.* and *Moe S.*
Et forenklet system for registrering av gingivitt hos tenåringer. Erfaringer etter tre års bruk i Oppegård kommune. Nor. Tannlægeforen. Tid., 1983: 93: 157–161.

25. *Hansen B. F., Bellini H. T.* and *Gjermo P.*
A multinational study on the prevalence of radiographic bone loss in young adults. 1983. (Manus)

26. *Hansen B. F., Gjermo P.* and *Bergwitz-Larsen R.*
Periodontal breakdown in 15-year-old Norwegians. J. Clin. Periodontol., 1984, 11: 125–131.

27. *Hansen, E. R.*
Evaluation of preventive programmes for school children. In Dental Health Care in Scandinavia. (Frandsen A. ed.) Quintessence, Berlin, 1982, pp 83–98.

28. *Hatle G.* and *Gjermo P.*
Effekten av klorhexidinholdig tannpasta på gingivalforholdene hos en gruppe utviklingshemmede. Tidsskr. Nor. Lægeforen., 1979, 99: 641–642.

29. *Hazen S. P.*
Indices for the measurement of gingival inflammation in clinical studies of oral hygiene and periodontal disease. J. Periodontal Res., 1974, 9: Suppl. 14, 61–71.

30. *Heløe L. A.*
Dental care delivery systems in Denmark, Finland, Norway and Sweden. In Dental Health Care in Scandinavia. (Frandsen A. ed.) Quintessence, Chicago, 1982, pp 11–20.

31. *Hoag P. M.*
Plaque control in the treatment of periodontitis. In Tissue Management in Restorative Dentistry. (Malone W. F. P. and Porter Z. C. eds.) John Wright, Psg Inc., London, 1982, pp 1–35.

32. *Hollender L., Lindhe J.* and *Koch G.*
A roentgenographic study of healthy and inflamed periodontal tissues in children. J. Periodontal. Res., 1966, 1: 146–151.

33. *Holm A. K.*
Evaluation of preventive programmes for preschool children. In Dental Health Care in Scandinavia. (Frandsen A. ed.) Quintessence, Berlin, 1982, pp 55–72.

34. *Hoover J. N., Ellegaard B.* and *Attstrøm R.*
Radiographic and clinical examination of periodontal status of first molars in 15–16-year-old Danish schoolchildren. Scand. J. Dent. Res., 1981, 89: 260–263.

35. *Hugoson A., Koch G.* and *Rylander H.*
Prevalence and distribution of gingivitis-periodontitis in children and adolescents. Swed. Dent. J., 1981, 5: 91–103.

36. *Johansen J. R.*
A Survey in Norway for Causes of Loss of Permanent Teeth and the Number of Teeth Remaining after Extraction. University of Oslo, Oslo 1970. Thesis, pp 1–168.

37. *Johansen J. R., Gjermo P.* and *Bellini H. T.*
A system to classify the need for periodontal treatment. Acta Odontol. Scand., 1973, 31: 297–305.

38. *Lennon M. A.* and *Davies R. M.*
Prevalence and distribution of alveolar bone loss in a population of 15-year-old schoolchildren. J. Clin. Periodontol., 1974, 1: 175–182.

39. *Löe H.*
The gingival index, the plaque index and the retention index system. J. Periodontol., 1967, 38, Suppl. 610–616.

40. *Löe H., Ånerud Å., Boysen H.* and *Smith M.*
The natural history of periodontal disease in man. The rate of periodontal destruction before 40 years of age. J. Periodontol., 1978, 49: 607–620.

132

41. *Löe H.* and *Silness J.*
Periodontal disease in pregnancy. I. Prevalence and severity. Acta Odontol. Scand., 1963, 21: 533–551.

42. *Löe H., Theilade E. & Jensen S. B.*
Experimental gingivitis in man. J. Periodontol. 1965, 36: 177–187.

43. *Mandel I. D.*
Indices for measurement of soft accumulations in clinical studies of oral hygiene and periodontal disease. J. Periodontal. Res., 1974, 9: Suppl. 14, 7–30.

44. *Murtomaa H.* and *Ainamo J.*
Conception of Finnish people about their periodontal situation. Community Dent. Oral Epidemiol., 1977, 5: 195–199.

45. *Parsby J. E.*
Communication and Behavioral Change. In Preventive Dentistry in Practice. (Frandsen A. ed.) Munksgaard, Copenhagen, 1976, pp 92–113.

46. *Perioåret*
Nor. Tannlægeforen. Tid., 1981, 91: 359–360.

47. *Russel A. L.*
The Geographical Distribution and Epidemiology of Periodontal Disease. National Institute of Dental Research, Bethesda, Md. 1960, WHO/DH/34.

48. *Saxén L.*
Prevalence of juvenile periodontitis in Finland. J. Clin. Periodontol., 1980, 7: 177–186.

49. *Søgaard A. J.*
Tannhelsevaner, kunnskaper og meninger blant 9. klassinger i Tromsø. Munnpleien, 1981, 64: 63–66.

50. *Søgaard A. J*
Har Perioåret hatt noen effekt? En vurdering av den publikumsrettede delen av periodontikampanjen. Nor. Tannlægeforen. Tid., 1984, 94: 5–11.

51. *Søgaard A. J.* and *Stenvik R.*
Har Perioåret hatt noen effekt? Norske tannlegers oppfatning av Perioåret. Nor. Tannlægeforen. Tid., 1983, 93: 9–12.

52. *Tolo K., Schenck K. & Brandtzæg P.*
Enzyme-linked immunosorbent assay for human IgG, IgA and IgM antibodies to antigens from anaerobic cultures of seven oral bacteria. J. Immunol. Methods, 1981, 45: 27–40.

53. *Waerhaug J.*
Epidemiology of Periodontal Disease. Review of literature. In World Workshop in Periodontics, (Ramfjord S. P., Kerr D. A. and Ash M. M. eds.) University of Michigan, Ann Arbor, 1966, pp 181–211.

54. *Wåler S. M.* and *Rölla G.*
Dårlig ånde – Foetor ex ore. Nor. Tannlægeforen. Tid., 1982, 92: 235–236.

55. World Health Organization. Epidemiology, Etiology and Prevention of Periodontal Disease. TRS 621, WHO, Geneva, 1978.

10. Minimum Number of Teeth Needed to Satisfy Functional and Social Demands

Arnd F. Käyser

The aim of this review is to:

- Evaluate concepts regarding the number of teeth necessary for man living in a modern society.
- Discuss the influence of a shortened dental arch on oral function.
- Make recommendations for public dental health care and research.

Introduction

The teeth in the human dentition can be divided according to their function, into aesthetic units – serving primarily for the aesthetic function – and occlusal units (OU) primarily required for a stable occlusion (Table 10.1).

A minimum number of teeth for those living in Western countries will include the aesthetic units. Furthermore, it will be shown that the minimum number of OU will, as a rule, also include the first premolar units. This means that the problem can be put in terms of how many OU are needed, or to what extent the dental arch can be reduced or shortened. A shortened dental arch (SDA) is a dentition with a reduction of OU (Fig. 10.1).

At first sight it might seem absurd to question the minimum number of needed teeth in the human dentition. After all, one does not discuss the minimum number of fingers on the hand. Central to the problem is the importance of the part of the body for survival and function of the individual, and its susceptibility to disease.

Evolution

In the evolution of the human race we can observe a change in oral function. The hands took over the grasping and touching functions of the snout.[8] Intelligence influenced chewing function by inventing and producing refined food.

Consequently modern man uses a fraction of his potential chewing force.[4] Communication has become a more important function of the masticatory apparatus than chewing. The dentition is in a state of hypofunction.

In nature, biological systems have the ability to adapt to a changing environment. The phylogenetic reduction of the jaws and teeth is an evolutionary mechanism

Table 10.1 Functional classification of the 14 pairs of antagonistic teeth.

Location	Name	Number
Front	Aesthetic unit	6
Premolar area	Occlusal unit (OU)	4
Molar area	Occlusal unit	4 (8)[1]
Total	Functional unit	14

[1] In premolar equivalents.

135

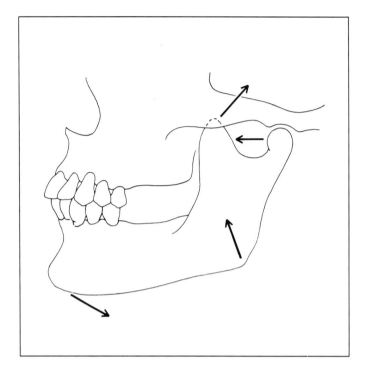

Fig. 10.1 A dental arch short-ened to the second premo-lars.

that may lag behind the environmental conditions in which humans live.[26]

One might question whether there is an optimal relationship between form and function in the dentition of modern man.[22] The problems of the third molar are well known. Their preventive removal is an ac-cepted procedure in dentistry.[1, 28, 42] With this procedure the number of functional units is reduced from 16 to 14 resulting in a SDA.

Oral Health and Minimum Number of Teeth

The natural dentition is frequently dam-aged by neglect, resulting in some form of mutilated dentition (Fig. 10.2). Caries and periodontal diseases may be considered

diseases of neglect.[11] Dentists can restore this mutilated dentition to a healthy func-tioning dentition. However, contrary to the desired aim, the restored dentition in most cases does not last the lifetime of the pa-tient.[34, 37] Neglect usually prevails. More-over, dental treatment, especially restora-tive treatment, has many negative side-ef-fects on the related tissues, the so-called biologic price.[43] Many studies have shown the high failure rate of traditional dental services.[9, 12, 24] Figure 10.2 illustrates that dental service is a never ending pro-cess.

Traditional dental services put emphasis on quantity at the expense of quality. Quantitative overtreatment does not guar-antee a healthy natural functioning denti-tion for life. Quality based on preventive measures, comes closer to that goal.[18, 30]

Traditional concepts and dogmas are re-

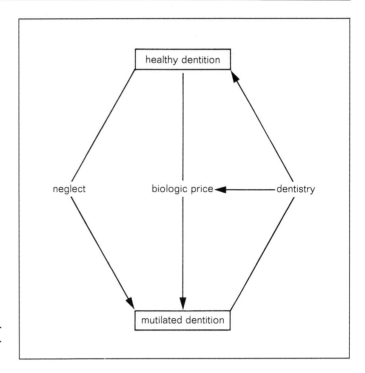

Fig. 10.2 Schematic repres- entation of the effect of tradi- tional dental service.

sponsible for the approaches leading to overtreatment.[27]

Influence of tooth loss on oral health

Hirschfeld stated in 1937[17] that a cause and effect chain of over eighty changes may result from the loss of a lower first permanent molar and that the loss of any other tooth in either arch may produce si- milar, if not quite so extensive, changes. Every individual tooth was considered to be a keystone, not only for one, but also for both dental arches. Failure to replace a missing tooth was said to result directly or indirectly in unlimited damage.

The dogma that missing teeth should be replaced as soon as possible can still be found in most prosthetic textbooks. Miss- ing a tooth is having a disease, according to *Ketterl*[25]: „das Lückengebiß ist eine

Krankheit. Der Zahnarzt ist zur Versor- gung verpflichtet, auch wenn der Patient eine systematische Vorbehandlung ablehnt." However, clinical observation shows that Hirschfeld's conclusions are questionable.

Karlsen[20] warned that missing teeth *per se* do not indicate prosthetic replacement. In 1974 *Ramfjord*[36] stated that "Replacement of lost molars is a common source of ia- trogenic periodontal disease, and should be avoided if requirements to aesthetics and functional stability can be satisfied without such replacements". He found that satisfactory function and occlusal, as well as neuromuscular stability, usually can be maintained if all anterior teeth and bicuspids are present, and that modern man's diet does not require an intact den- tition to meet functional demands. Clinical studies tend to support those observa- tions. Based on a literature review, *Pilot*[33]

Table 10.2 Estimation of the minimum number of teeth needed to satisfy functional demands of modern man.

Oral function	Needed teeth
Biting	12 front teeth
	4 premolars?
Chewing	8 premolars
	4 Molars?
Speech	12 front teeth
Aesthetics	12 front teeth
	4 upper premolars
Mandibular stability	12 front teeth
(mandibular comfort)	8 premolars
	4 molars?
Total	12 front teeth
	8 premolars
	4 molars (?)

Table 10.3 Possible effects of a SDA on the quality of oral function (effect: +, no effect: −).

Function	Effect
1. Start of digestion	
biting	−
tasting	−
chewing	+
swallowing	−
2. Communication	
speech	−
physiognomy	−
aesthetics	+
3. Occlusion (stability)	
residual dentition	+
TMJ	+
4. Parafunction	
bruxism	?

concluded that there is no scientific data available supporting the prosthetic restoration of SDA.

The effect of tooth loss depends on a combination of local and systemic factors (Fig. 10.3). Local factors include location and number of lost teeth, interarch relationship of remaining teeth, position of the tongue and presence of plaque. Systemic factors involve host resistance to disease, adaptive capacity, and age. The mode of action of the local factors is better known and understood than the systemic factors. Therefore the effects of tooth loss are just partly predictable. Extractions leading to interrupted dental arches generally seem to result in more negative effects than extractions leading to SDA.

The patient's appreciation of the dentition is different to that of the dentist. The patients needs teeth for appearance, chewing and oral comfort. The dentist, however, adds another item: a good occlusion, whatever that may mean. Table 10.2 shows the minimum number of teeth needed to satisfy functional demands.

The minimum number of teeth comes close to 12 front teeth and 8 premolars. A reduction beyond this number results in a SDA with impaired oral function, both in quality and in quantity (Table 10.3, Fig. 10.4)

The loss of molar support has been related to functional disturbances of the temporomandibular joint.[10, 39] Now it is considered just one of the possible aetiological factors.[6] Some studies report a correlation between the number of residual teeth and mandibular dysfunction.[5]

Occlusal concepts

The traditional, mechanically orientated occlusal concepts for a healthy dentition used to stress the morphological requirements of complete dental arches (Angle concept, gnathology, Pankey-Mann-Schuyler concept). Molar support, in relation to the temporomandibular joint, was considered to be of prime importance. Now the trend is toward functional requirements

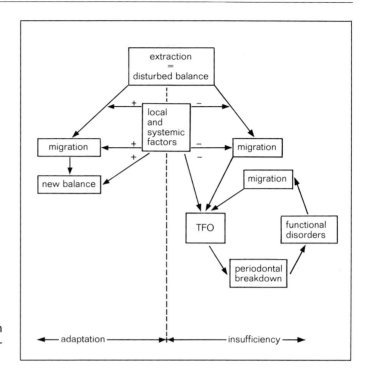

Fig. 10.3 The effects of tooth loss on the remaining dentition.

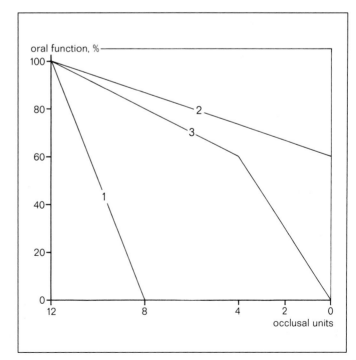

Fig. 10.4 The theoretical relationships between oral function and shortened dental arches. Occlusal units = pairs of antagonistic posteriors expressed in premolar equivalents.

1. Absence of adaptive capacity (Hirschfeld[17])
2. Presence of adaptive capacity (Ramfjord[36])
3. Adaptive capacity until a certain number of occlusal units.

such as mandibular stability, satisfactory aesthetics, oral comfort and the absence of pathology.[15, 35, 36] The minimum number of teeth may vary from individual to individual.

Studies on Reduced Dentitions

Studies under controlled conditions on the function of reduced dentitions are scarce. Most information dates from 1975 and after, and is derived from cross-sectional studies.

A cross-sectional investigation was carried out in Holland on the changes in oral functions in SDA.[21, 23] The investigated subjects were selected from the patients who attended the restorative and prosthetic departments of the dental school in Nijmegen. The total number was 118, of which 90 had a SDA for more than 2 years and 28 subjects were in possession of a complete dentition (control group). The ages varied between 19 and 71 years. In 82% of the subjects the shortened dental condition existed for more than 5 years. The subjects were classified into six classes, according to the degree and the symmetry of the shortened dentition. The length of the dental arch in the premolar-molar area was expressed in occlusal units (OU), i.e. pairs of occluding posterior teeth, 1 molar unit being considered equal to 2 premolar units. Class I represents the control group (11–12 OU), classes IIa and IIb the asymmetric, and classes IIIa and IIIb the symmetric groups (a and b indicate the number of OU). Class IV is the extremely shortened group (0–2 OU; Fig. 10.5).

On examination the subjects were questioned, representative teeth and radiographs were scored and the subjects submitted to a chewing test. The representative teeth used were teeth numbers 1, 2, and 3 from the maxilla and the teeth numbers 4, 5, and 6 from the premolar-molar

area in the lower jaw. The influence of the SDA on the remaining dentition was assessed using the following variables: alveolar bone height, interdental contact relation within the dental arch, attrition, overbite of the anteriors 21 and 31, and contact between the anteriors of upper and lower jaw in habitual occlusion (intercuspal position). The effects on the temporomandibular joint were investigated by recording the presence or absence of the three main features of mandibular dysfunction. These are:

1. Pain in the region of the joints and/or the masticatory muscles.
2. Limited opening of the mouth.
3. Joint sounds.

The appearance of the remaining dentition was assessed by the patient. The results of the chewing tests showed a highly significant correlation between masticatory capacity and number of OU. With decreasing numbers of OU the numbers of chewing strokes needed for swallowing increased. In asymmetrically shortened dental arches chewing is done unilaterally on the side of the longer arch, and in extremely shortened arches it is done with the front teeth. The subjects started complaining about their masticatory function when the number of OU was less than 4 in symmetrically SDA and less than 6 in asymmetrically shortened arches.

The remaining dentition showed that in all shortened classes the number of tooth contacts between the anterior teeth in habitual occlusion was higher and the number of interdental contacts in the premolar area was smaller than in class I. In class IV cases the alveolar bone height was less, the number of interdental contacts in the upper anterior area was less and the attrition in the upper anterior area higher. The decrease in bone height was partly due to age and partly to the effect of the shortened dental arch. More complaints in the masticatory muscles were found in subjects chewing with their front

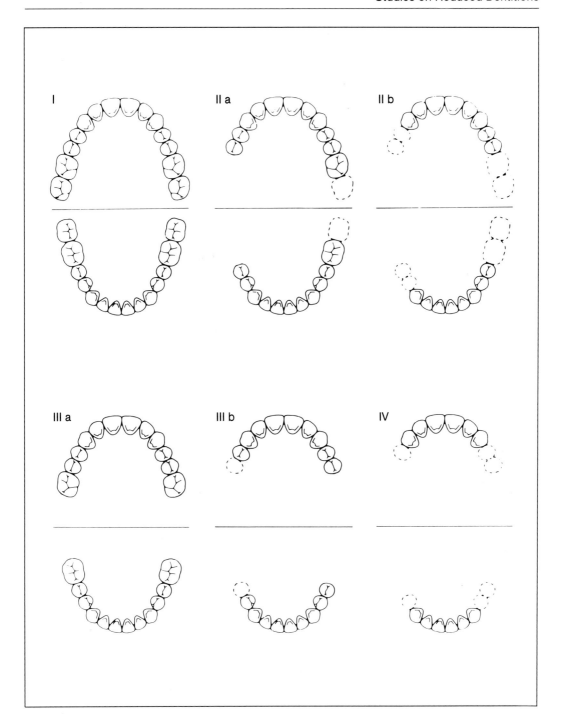

Fig. 10.5   Schematic representation of the six classes showing variation in occlusal units within the classes.

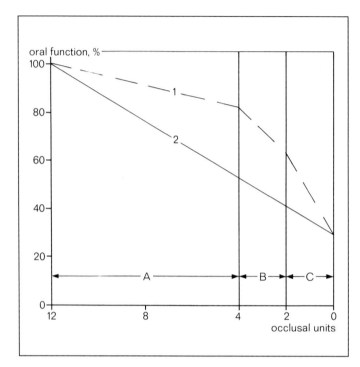

Fig. 10.6 The relationship between oral function and shortened dental arches.

1. Adaptive capacity until 4 occlusal units.
2. Progressively decreasing adaptive capacity.
   (A) area of sufficient oral function;
   (B) turning range;
   (C) area of insufficient oral function.

teeth. No correlation was found between temporomandibular joint problems and unilateral chewing.

A SDA in the lower jaw did not raise appreciable aesthetic problems. In the upper jaw a shortening until the second premolar might result in a negative but acceptable evaluation of the appearance. The first and second premolar have an important aesthetic function: if one of these two teeth is missing the result is a negative appraisal of the aesthetic situation and the subject may want prosthetic replacement. The number of complaints rose as the number of OU decreased (32% of the subjects in class IV complained about deficiencies in relation to aesthetics and chewing capacity). The results are summarized in Figure 10.6. Two patterns can be distinguished in the observed change in oral functions:

1. Oral functions that change slowly until 4 occlusal units remain and then change rapidly (alveolar bone height, aesthetics, interdental contact, muscular activity).
2. Oral functions that change progressively with changes in numbers of OU (chewing capacity, contact between the anterior teeth in habitual occlusion).

The correlation between masticatory capacity and number of OU is in agreement with the results of *Helkimo et al.*[16] though different methods were used. The differences in contact relation of the teeth (interdental contact within the arch and contact of the upper and lower anteriors) are an indication of adaptive migration, which takes place in the remaining dentition (Fig. 10.7). This migration is not necessarily deleterious to the dentition. The bound-

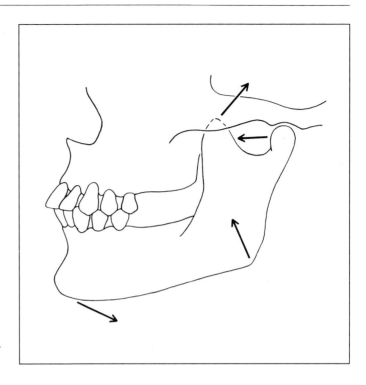

Fig. 10.7 Migration in a shortened dental arch.

ary between physiological adaptation and pathological effect is difficult to define. Only in the extremely shortened class IV was the alveolar bone height less than in the other classes. The importance of the aesthetic function of the upper premolars is in agreement with the findings of *Silness*[38] and *Valderhaug* and *Karlsen*[41] concerning the location and distribution of fixed partial dentures. The results lead to the assumption that for a number of oral functions a critical range exists in which they change rapidly. This range is located between 2 and 4 OU (Fig. 10.6). Based on these results the tentative conclusion is that there is sufficient adaptive capacity in SDA when at least 4 occlusal units are left, preferably in a symmetrical position. This conclusion is now tested in Nijmegen in a longitudinal study using the same method. Several other studies confirmed the above

mentioned results. Reports of the *Nyman* and *Lindhe* team[31, 32] indicate that the number of teeth is not the decisive factor for successful results. Periodontal tissue area may be reduced as long as it is kept in a healthy condition.[31, 32]

Haraldson[14] studied SDA in a situation where they were created artificially. He investigated the oral function in 35 patients provided with osseointegrated implant bridges in one or both jaws. In 85% of these subjects the functional occlusion was extended to the second premolars. The results showed objective and subjective satisfactory function with regard to biting force, chewing efficiency, EMG activity and oral comfort.

Grunder and *Imperiali*[13] investigated a group of 300 Swiss citizens. In the age group of 50–59 years they found 60% persons with SDA. Only 50% of these

143

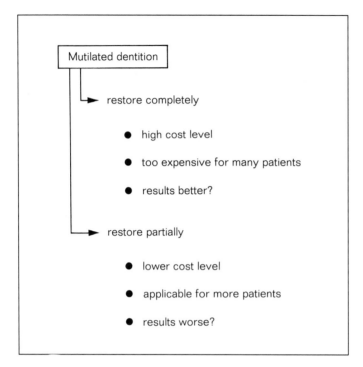

Fig. 10.8 Different strategies to restore a mutilated dentition.

subjects had prosthetic appliances made to extend the SDA. Of this last group, again only 50% used their prosthesis. There were no complaints raised about impaired oral function. Only 3% of the 300 subjects indicated restricted chewing comfort.

In an epidemiologic study on 750 subjects in Holland, *Battistuzzi*[3] found no correlation between the number of missing posteriors (premolars and molars) and the subjective function of the masticatory system.

Conclusions

Based on clinical observation, as well as research findings, it can be stipulated that the minimum number of teeth varies individually and depends on local and system-ic factors. Spatial relationship between the lower and upper teeth, age, adaptive capacity and occlusal activity are important factors. Current information suggests that the minimum number of teeth is 20 (6 aesthetic units and 4 premolar occlusal units) for subjects over approximately 45 years, with moderate occlusal activity. For younger subjects and in those cases with pronounced occlusal activity, the minimum number is 24 (6 aesthetic units, 4 premolar OU and 2 molar OU).

The suggested minimum number of teeth and their location coincide roughly with the general pattern of tooth loss in European populations, with the exception of the first molar.[3, 13, 19, 40] This is not surprising as the fate of teeth is influenced not only by dental diseases, but also by the functional evaluation of teeth and its consequences in the motivation to save or to extract them.[33]

In planning dental health service it should be realized that the aim of maintaining a healthy natural functioning dentition for life, does not imply saving a maximum number of teeth. This goal may be reached more predictably if the emphasis is put on quality and not quantity, particularly in terms of preventive and maintenance programmes.[2, 18] Figure 10.8 shows two different strategies which may be used to restore a diseased or mutilated dentition. Many dental health care systems still promote quantity treatment without evaluation of the results. This may lead to overtreatment, rising cost levels and ultimately to failure of the system. Much time and effort is spent on molar teeth, which in spite of the efforts seem to be lost prematurely.[29]

Problem-solving approaches should be incorporated in public health strategies. This means that treatment should only be implemented in cases where the existing condition leads to relevant problems. The treatment should be aimed at solving those problems and not primarily at restoring morphologic ideals, especially in groups at high risk to dental disease.

Recommendations

1. The suggested conclusions should be verified in longitudinal studies.
2. Public dental health programmes should implement existing research findings in order to be effective at controllable cost levels.
3. Strategies for treatment planning should be screened and, if necessary, adjusted in order to:

   (a) concentrate time and effort primarily on strategic teeth;
   (b) promote problem-solving approaches in occlusal therapy instead of traditional morphologic based approaches;

   (c) control the provision of expensive treatments based on patient cooperation and effective quality control.

DeVan concluded in 1952[7]: 'Our objective should be the perpetual preservation of what remains rather than meticulous restoration of what is missing'. After 30 years this statement is still valid, often cited but seldom put into practice. With our present knowledge it can be adjusted as follows:

Our objective should be *preservation of the strategic part of the remaining dentition*, rather than the meticulous restoration of what is damaged or missing.

References

1. *Ash M. M.*
   Third molars as periodontal problems. Dent. Clin. North. Amer., 1964, 8: 51–61.

2. *Axelsson P.* and *Lindhe J.*
   Effect of controlled oral hygiene procedures on caries and periodontal disease in adults – Results after 6 years. J. Clin. Periodontol., 1981, 8: 239–248.

3. *Battistuzzi P. G. F. C. M.*
   Het gemutileerde gebit. Thesis, University of Nijmegen, 1982.

4. *Carlsson G. E.*
   Bite force and chewing efficiency. In Frontiers of Oral Physiology. Vol. 1, (Kawamura, Y., ed.) Karger, Basel etc. 1974, pp. 265–292.

5. *Carlsson G. E., Kopp S.* and *Öberg T.*
   Arthritis and allied diseases of the temporomandibular joint. In Temporomandibular Joint, Function and Dysfunction. (Zarb, G.A. and Carlsson, G.E., eds.) Munksgaard, Copenhagen, 1979, pp. 269–320.

6. *De Boever J. A.*
   Functional disturbances of the temporomandibular joint. In Temporomandibular Joint, Function and Dysfunction. (Zarb, G. A. and Carlsson, G.E., eds.) Munksgaard, Copenhagen, 1979, pp. 193–214.

7. *DeVan M. M.*
   The nature of the partial denture foundation: suggestions for its preservation. J. Prosthet. Dent., 1952, 2: 210–218.

8. *Du Brul E. L.*
Origin and evolution of the oral apparatus. In: Frontiers of Oral Physiology. Vol. 1, (Kawamura, Y., ed.) Karger, Basel etc. 1974, pp. 1–30.

9. *Elderton R. J.*
The prevalence of failure of restorations. J. Dent., 1976, 4: 207–210.

10. *Gerber A.*
Kiefergelenk und Zahnokklusion. Dtsch. zahnärztl. Z., 1971, 26: 119–141.

11. *Glickman I.*
Clinical Periodontology. 4th edn. Saunders, Philadelphia, 1972, pp. 444.

12. *Going R. E.* and *Jendresen M. D.*
Failures related to materials used in restorative dentistry. Dent. Clin. North. Amer., 1972, 16: 71–86.

13. *Grunder M.* and *Imperiali D.*
Zahnarztbesuch und Informationsgrad zur Prophylaxe, Mundhygienegewohnheiten, zahnärztliche Versorgung und subjektive Kaufähigkeit bei sozio-ökonomisch unterschiedlichen Bevölkerungsschichten in der Schweiz. Thesis, University of Bern, 1982.

14. *Haraldson T.*
Functional evaluation of bridges on osteointegrated Implants in the edentulous jaw. Thesis, University of Göteborg, 1979.

15. *Hedegard B.* and *Landt H.*
Die Entwicklung von Behandlungs-Konzepten. Zahnärztl. Welt Rundschau, Reform, 1982, 91: 40–43.

16. *Helkimo E., Carlsson G. E.* and *Helkimo M.*
Chewing efficiency and state of dentition. Acta Odontol. Scand., 1978, 36: 33–41.

17. *Hirschfeld I.*
The individual missing tooth. J. Amer. Dent. Assoc., 1937, 24: 67–82.

18. *Hugoson A.* and *Koch G.*
Oral health in 1000 individuals aged 3–10 years in the community of Jönköping, Sweden. Swed. Dent. J., 1979, 3: 69–87.

19. *Johansen J. R.*
A survey in Norway for causes of loss of permanent teeth and the number of teeth remaining after extraction. Thesis, University of Oslo, 1970.

20. *Karlsen, K.*
Factors that influence the provision of partial prosthetic appliances. J. Dent., 1973, 1: 52–57.

21. *Käyser, A. F.*
De gebitsfuncties bij verkorte tandbogen, Thesis, University of Nijmegen, 1976.

22. *Käyser A. F.*
Clinical aspects of shortened dental arches. Proceedings of the European Prosthodontic Association. 3rd Annual Meeting. Glumslöv, Sweden, 1979.

23. *Käyser A. F.*
Shortened dental arches and oral function, J. Oral Rehabil., 1981, 8: 457–462.

24. *Kerschbaum T.* and *Voss R.*
Die praktische Bewährung von Krone und Inlay. Dtsch. Zahnärztl. Z., 1981, 36: 243–249.

25. *Ketterl W.*
Die Vorbereitung des parodontal-geschädigten Gebisses für eine prothetische Versorgung. Zahnärztl. Welt Rundschau, Reform, 1979, 88: 715–716.

26. *Kraus B. S., Jordan R. J.* and *Abrams L.*
Dental Anatomy and Occlusion. Williams and Wilkins, Baltimore, 1969, pp. 291–293.

27. *Lang N. P.*
Was heißt funktionelle Rekonstruktion im parodontal reduzierten Gebiß. Schweiz Monatschr. Zahnheilkd., 1982, 92: 365–377.

28. *Lytle J. J.*
Indications and contraindications for removal of the impacted tooth. Dent. Clin. North. Amer., 1979, 23: 333–346.

29. *Meeuwissen R.* and *Eschen S.*
Twintig jaar tandheelkundige zorg: verhoogt tandboogverkorting effectiviteit en kwaliteit van de zorg? Tandheelkundig Jaar, 1982: 23–30.

30. *Mühlemann, H. R.*
Zum Wandel der Zahnheilkunde. Schweiz Monatsschr. Zahnheilkd., 1979, 89: 998–1003.

31. *Nyman S.* and *Lindhe J.*
Prosthetic rehabilitation of patients with advanced periodontal disease. J. Clin. Periodontol., 1976, 3: 135–147.

32. *Nyman S.* and *Ericsson I.*
The capacity of reduced periodontal tissues to support fixed bridgework. J. Clin. Periodontol., 1982: 9: 409–414.

33. *Pilot T.*
Pleidooi tegen het verlengen van de verkorte tandboog. Ned. Tijdschr. Tandheelkd., 1978, 85: 477–480.

34. *Pilot, T.*
Analysis of the overall effectiveness of treatment of periodontal disease. In: Efficacy of Treatment Procedures in Periodontics. (Shanley D. ed.) Quintessence, Chicago, 1980, pp. 213–231.

35. *Ramfjord S. P.* and *Ash M. M.*
Occlusion, 3rd edn. Saunders, Philadelphia, 1983 pp. 157–168.

36. *Ramfjord S. P.*
Periodontal aspects of restorative dentistry. J. Oral Rehabil., 1974, 1: 107–126.

37. *Sheiham A.*
An evaluation of the success of dental care in the United Kingdom. Brit. Dent. J., 1973, 135: 271–279.

38. *Silness, J.*
Distribution of artificial crowns and fixed partial dentures. J. Prosthet. Dent., 1970, 23: 641–647.

39. *Steinhardt, G.*
Über die gegenseitige Abhängigkeit zwischen Paradentium und Kiefergelenk beim Kauvorgang. Dtsch. Zahnärztl. Z., 1950: 5: 1157–1173.

40. *Todd J. E.* and *Walker A. M.*
Adult Dental Health, Vol. 1, England and Wales 1968–1978. HMSO, London, 1980, pp. 35–41.

41. *Valderhaug J.* and *Karlsen K.*
Frequency and location of artificial crowns and fixed partial dentures constructed at a dental school. J. Oral Rehabil., 1976, 3: 75–81.

42. Workshop National Institute of Dental Research. NIH consensus development conference for removal of third molars. J. Oral Surg., 1980, 38: 235–236.

43. *Zarb G. A., Bergman B., Clayton J. A.* and *Mackay H. F.*
Prosthodontic Treatment for Partially Edentulous Patients. Mosby, St. Louis, 1978, pp. 56–62.

11. Dental Health Education and Periodontal Disease: Health Policies, Disease Trends, Target Groups and Strategies

Michael Craft

Introduction

'The prevention and control of periodontal disease presents a serious challenge to the profession. The British Society of Periodontology has expressed the view that it is totally unrealistic and unnecessary to aim for zero plaque and zero gingival inflammation in the population at large. A more realistic aim would be the life-long maintenance of a dentition which is functional, socially acceptable and does not pose a threat to the general health of the individual.

This aim requires an expansion of programmes of dental health education. The objectives should be to motivate and encourage the public to achieve and maintain a high standard of oral hygiene thereby reducing plaque levels and reversing and controlling the disease process. A high standard of oral hygiene is the only effective primary preventive measure currently available against periodontal disease' (from *Towards Better Dental Health*).[55]

As this Workshop on Periodontal Disease meets, the above extract is already 12 months old. Despite many recent national reports relating prevention and health, this is the only one to place a major emphasis on the problems posed by periodontal disease. Yet despite growing concern, no action has so far been taken to implement its recommendations.

This review looks at the place of dental health education (DHE) in the control of periodontal disease, before considering national health spending and disease trends, current DHE work with target groups; future plans for extension of this work, including a coordinated national preventive strategy.

Disease Prevention

During the last 5 years in the UK, a broad concensus has begun to emerge over the need for prevention of disease. Several expert committees and a Royal Commission have reported on aspects of health services, and all have placed emphasis on prevention in general, and dental disease in particular.[3, 15, 17, 44, 45, 46, 48, 55] Yet, in general, the emphasis on the prevention of periodontal disease remains weak. In fact, it is necessary to turn to the scientific literature to discover the true dimensions of the problem and the well-accepted research that allows us to predict the strong relationships between effective oral hygiene and periodontal disease, especially in its early stages.[4, 5, 6, 28, 36, 47, 51]

Priority of Periodontal Disease

Perhaps, therefore, the first stage in considering the role of DHE in the prevention of periodontal disease must be the recognition of the dominance hitherto occupied by dental caries; a dominance that may be historically related to the emergence of a craft profession responding to the acute sufferings of its increasingly sugar-dependent clients. This social process may have been reinforced by the chronic nature of periodontal disease and the perception of its early symptoms, such as bleeding, as insignificant and normal,[18] a situation not helped by the fact that only some 46% of the population visit a dentist for routine treatment.[54] The popular priority given to periodontal problems will be influenced by a combination of cultural patterns, social networks and economic conditions. This complex process is dynamic and recent evidence amongst adolescents, for example, shows increased existing knowledge concerning plaque and the function of toothbrushing, as well as positive attitudes towards dental health.[21, 23]

However, consider, for example, the pressures of redundancy and unemployment (with associated health problems), large families, low income, rising prices and high interest rates, poor living conditions. Then combine these with lack of emotional and social resources, patterns of early marriage, social isolation and the stigma of poverty.[13] In such situations, to attribute the possibility of choice in health matters is to assume a degree of control over the environment which does not stand up to enquiry. Yet in Europe, 30 million people (10 million households), might be classed as living in such conditions of poverty.[14]

The Situational Context

Against this background, therefore, a basic assumption in any attempt to prevent periodontal disease through DHE will be the recognition of its low public (and, to a lesser extent, professional) priority and the need to avoid any tendency to blame

the victim of social and economic circumstances for the disease problem, as distinct from concentrating on the circumstances themselves.[31, 50] Such an approach does not rule out changes at the individual level – it merely renders DHE strategies more realistic, more effective and less disappointing. This approach will also serve to ensure the importance of relevant objectives against which to carry out meaningful evaluation; of choosing discrete population segments that are grouped by similar patterns of beliefs, behaviour and risk to disease that are investigated and defined prior to intervention.[52, 53] How, then, can programmes of DHE be designed and carried out to overcome this considerable hurdle? To answer this question it is first necessary to consider the political and health context within which such programmes are now required. What trends can be observed, both in health policies and in disease trends, that are relevant and likely to influence the incidence and prevalence of periodontal disease and our response?

Health Spending and Disease Trends

Evidence now exists that suggests health spending may soon undergo severe and prolonged limitation, whether in terms of inadequate inflation-proofing or actual cutback. Since the beginning of this century, health spending (percentage of gross national product) in the major EEC countries has risen from 1% to approximately 7% up until 1980, but is now likely to stabilize and fall.[42] This pattern may be traced to the virtual end of optimism in the overall control of disease that was exemplified in the World Health Organisation definition of health as 'a state of complete physical, mental and social wellbeing'. This is now widely regarded as unattainable. We may also be witnessing the start of economic and philosophical retrenchment in attitudes to health care. Certainly many governments are concerned about the 5% rise in such spending since the Second World War and, in more general terms, much of this spending has received powerful criticism as being misdirected and unnecessary.[12, 32, 38] Whilst inequalities of health services and variations in mortality are still far too great,[30] variations in the subjective meaning of health – such as impairment, disability and handicap – are now more accepted in normality, and perhaps this is welcome. However, in the UK, a new crisis of resources has been superimposed on this shifting pattern and which may spell the end of the post-war boom in health care. Whilst the National Health Service (NHS) needs additional resources each year merely to continue at its present level, the Government is calling for widespread economies. The result has been a spate of reports at the highest levels in the Service and from all parts of the UK, forecasting drastic reductions in service. It has even been suggested that plans exist to abolish the NHS in its present form, and many observers expect that any reductions will affect mainly the most vulnerable groups: the young, the elderly, the handicapped, the poor.[33] Under the NHS reorganization of 1982, community dental services (as distinct from general practice) have emerged with lowered morale and impaired functions in many regions. Despite wide evidence of falling caries rates, there is real concern about the effects these impairments will have upon high risk groups who normally make most use of these services, and often make little use of preventive services. Indeed, it may be significant that evidence from the USA suggests that the fall in caries is not uniform and remains high in poorer, black communities,[1, 29] and, in any case, the reasons for the change, welcome as it is, are not yet clear.[40]

A Periodontal Epidemic?

The failure of the British National Health Service to contain its costs has been traced by many observers to the emergence of chronic disease in the wake of acute conditions. As *Lord Wade* commented in his book 'Europe and the British Health Service':[56]

'That the future was not clearly foreseen is, no doubt, understandable. Attention was concentrated on getting rid of the most obvious and most acute diseases. It was not appreciated that by eliminating them or lessening their severity, more time would have to be devoted to chronic disabilities which would require more continuous care. There were few who foresaw that greater longevity would bring with it a multitude of disorders associated with old age'.

A similar situation could now occur following the fall in caries, resulting in an increase in both the incidence and prevalence of periodontal disease. Four main reasons may be advanced for this prediction:

1. The dentate population of the UK is predicted to rise to about 85% by the year 2020,[8] and this process may be accelerated by the falling caries rate. In fact, the same source estimates a 40% to 50% increase in numbers of teeth at risk. This increase in standing teeth may mean more associated periodontal pockets, lesions and problems resulting from destructive restorative treatment. This may occur at all ages, but particularly amongst the older age groups.[9] There are 7.5 million people aged 65 or over in the UK. As a whole, this group is already grossly lacking in social support and is not even likely to be accessible for periodontal therapy.
2. Evidence is accumulating that, amongst adolescents, school meals uptake is falling and that snackbased meals (including sweets) are eaten increasingly,

both in and out of school.[7, 26, 39] It is also suggested that poorer children are worst affected.[10] This tendency might lead not only to increased plaque accumulations, but possibly to higher frequencies of sucrose intake and a return of caries.

3. Periodontal disease is believed to begin in adolescence at about the age of 15[11, 34] and for a variety of social and health reasons young adults (and especially males) are at higher risk of dental disease.[19] Recently, charges for dental treatment were extended to those aged 18 or over and, thus, many more may be deterred from seeking treatment and placed even more at risk.

4. There is a continued predominance of the medical model in health service provision, in which it is implied that the main determinants of health and illness are essentially biological, uncontaminated by the wider social and economic environment.[27] As a consequence, the solutions to problems such as dental disease, are seen largely within the framework laid down by this model – the continued search for an anti-caries vaccine is one example of this approach. Thus, a fall in caries may be seen by society as evidence only of successful and objective engineering. Beliefs, attitudes and economic circumstances may be thought to be irrelevant and a regression of positive dental attitudes could, therefore, occur. Why bother to find alternatives to sugar, or brush effectively when dental science has succeeded in conquering the scourge of dental disease by other, more convenient means?

All these assumptions concerning the possibility of an approaching epidemic of periodontal disease may prove to be incorrect, and the only evidence available is conflicting; Anderson[2] reported gingival improvement (in relation to caries reduction) and surveys in the USA show positive trends.[1] However, despite lowered prevalence, severity remains unchanged and large increases in the disease have appeared in non-white populations.[29] But it is hard to avoid the conclusion that this eventuality is at least worthy of consideration, and raises serious questions about the appropriate response. If the socio-economic determinants of periodontal disease are considered important, then DHE is central in any European strategy for prevention.

Current United Kingdom National Programmes of DHE

In the UK, four rival toothpaste manufactures are active in the field of DHE, providing materials to particular age groups of the school population, but mainly amongst 5 to 10-year-olds. Although some attention is being paid to evaluation, the DHE campaigns of these companies are an integral part of their overall industrial aims and there is no doubt that their contribution to DHE is significant. However, it is not possible to say how significant, since nothing has been published concerning the reception or effectiveness of these programmes.

In contrast, the Government-funded Health Education Council Dental Health Study has, since 1975, researched, developed and tested two successful programmes for target groups at high risk: children (3 to 5-years-old) and adolescents (13 to 14-years-old). This work is the only published and evaluated work on a national scale and the field trials held are believed to be the largest of their kind in Europe.

The 'Natural Nashers' programme

The 'Natural Nashers' programme for 13 to 14-year-olds is now being nationally disseminated through District Dental Officers, since it is directly relevant to preventing periodontal disease which begins in adolescence. The description given here is a general one – detailed evaluation results have been published elsewhere.[20, 21, 22, 23, 24] By 1984 it will have been used by 70.000 pupils in 200 schools.

'Natural Nashers' has been developed with due regard to relevant experiences from the disciplines of medical sociology education and curriculum development, as well as dental health education. It is intended for use with 13 to 14-year-old adolescents in secondary schools – a relatively untouched group where increasing rates of dental disease are matched by important features of secondary socialization (the influence of peer and reference groups, grooming behaviour, change and modification of roles). It is 3 weeks in length (with additional optional project work) and is designed to be integrated into the third-year biology curriculum, using three 70 to 80 minute sessions. Each session contain a key lesson (slide presentation of information), a class experiment (activity and participation) and pupil worksheets (reinforcement). The content of the programme includes (1) the concept and nature of bacterial plaque, how to see it (disclosing) and how to remove it (effective brushing); and (2) the aetiology of dental decay and gum disease. The programme as a whole, whilst resting upon the distinction of prevention from cure, aims to promote self-care rather than resort to professional therapy. In recognition of home influences, each child receives a personal dental health kit and takes home a special diary of activities (recording personal plaque removal, counting teeth of brothers and sisters, monitoring the diet and interviewing family members). The desirability of activity in learning dictates the necessity of challenging classroom experiments to allow for peer working relationships and the release of anxiety.

Along with raising the priority of dental health and recognising the importance of the home, an emphasis is placed on choice and decision-making in health and the discovery of existing expertise. It is hoped that the target group approach, along with the inclusion of these situational factors and integration into the curriculum, will successfully combine to avoid victim blaming.

Integration into the curriculum is achieved through the use of an initial workshop (using a comprehensive teachers guide) to brief teachers, and negotiate variations. Emphasis is placed upon not changing the teacher's normal role. Each teacher is assigned a fieldworker, whose role is to assist teachers, minimise variation and provide evaluative data. Teachers are provided with slides, overhead transparencies and a comprehensive guide, whilst each pupil receives a folder of materials (worksheets, experiment sheets, stickers and leaflets, a home activities diary and a home care kit). The materials developed in conjunction with teachers, and written at two ability levels, are designed to be part of the normal biology curriculum (rather than a separate dental health input). The materials make provision for comprehension of concepts and reinforcement of the message and are produced in-house to high standards. This helps to contain costs, whilst allowing for rapid modification, updating and variation for local need – such as language translation.

The trials of the programme in 1980/81, ran among 6700 pupils in 45 largely urban, mixed sex, state comprehensive schools in England and Scotland. A quasi-experimental control group design was used and evaluation was carried out at the levels of *process* (teachers questionnaires, pupils worksheets, fieldworkers reports) and *outcome* (pupils' pre- and postquestionnaires, worksheets, plaque and gingival scores), amongst a random sub-sample (n = 1900) divided between study (n = 1300) and control (n = 600). Eighty-

Table 11.1 Longterm changes in plaque and gingival scores (whole mouth averages). "Natural Nashers" implementation trials.

	1 Pl	1 Gi	2 Pl	2 Gi	3 Pl	3 Gi	4 Pl	4 Gi	5 Pl	5 Gi	6 Pl	6 Gi
T1[1]	13.6	8.6	15.2	9.3	15.3	10.4	17.1	12.7	13.2	12.5	14.8	11.0
T2[1]	7.1	8.0	10.9	10.5	14.9	9.8	16.2	12.0	11.8	10.9	13.4	11.0
T3[2]	12.9	10.7	15.6	10.9	14.5	10.4	14.9	11.4	13.1	10.8	15.7	11.6
T4[3]	11.1	8.9	11.9	10.4	12.8	10.8	12.0	11.2	10.9	10.1	13.3	11.4
n =	22		22		31		29		21		20	

[1] Schools 1,2 – Feb. 4–15, March 13–21, 1980
  Schools 3,4 – March 24–April 2, May 5–16, 1980
  Schools 5,6 – May 19–23, June 23–27, 1980
[2] All schools – Nov. 19–21, 1980
[3] All schools – Dec. 10–12, 1980

three teachers completed a questionnaire and 330 fieldworkers' reports were analysed. Two hundred and fifty pupils were further examined after a minimum of 6 months.

An average 59% of pupils were from manual occupation backgrounds, with substantial ethnic minorities. Average DMF at baseline was 6.

Clinical outcomes were measured (pre and post) using the Löe Plaque Index[37] and the Cowell Gingival Index.[16] Reductions in plaque levels averaged 20% and gingival inflammation 9%.

Large gains in knowledge and attitudes were recorded. For example, gains of 55–60% on the importance of sugar frequency, and 40–50% increases in self-care beliefs. In contrast, baseline levels of knowledge concerning plaque and reasons for toothbrushing ranged from 60–85% and at these high levels only small gains were made.

A longer term follow-up was conducted in several schools (after 6 months) and gingival scores recorded before (T3) and after a short reinforcement programme (T4). As Table 11.1 shows, the significant difference in inflammation-free ($GI = 0$) margins between T1 and T2 (i. e. after the initial programme) was maintained after 6 months (T3).

Despite the fall in inflammation free margins after 6 months (14.4% at T3), a further significant increase was observed after a very brief reinforcement programme – consistent with the investigators' view that reinforcement is undoubtedly necessary. However, the figures given for T3 and T4 are the means for six schools, and a fuller picture of changes shows that the original reductions in gingival inflammation or plaque levels after the initial programme were maintained in three schools and that the average reduction in plaque levels after the reinforcement was 16%.

Other data from a subsequent trial in Scotland[23] in 1981 amongst 1500 pupils, concerning longterm effectiveness of 'Natural Nashers' shows that plaque scores in the

Table 11.2 Frequency distribution of plaque index scores zero and two plus for study and control groups, short- and longterm.

	Study		Control	
	PlI = 0 (%)	PlI = 2+ (%)	PlI = 0 (%)	PlI = 2+ (%)
All surfaces				
Baseline	2	61	6	51
5 weeks	8	36	6	49
28 weeks	1	52	4	54
Incisors				
Baseline	3	40	14	18
5 weeks	16	20	14	29
28 weeks	13	32	8	37
Molars				
Baseline	0	86	0	84
5 weeks	0	59	0	74
28 weeks	0	60 .	0	79

study group sample (n = 216) were significantly lower than the control group (n = 194) both after the initial programme (P<0.01) and after 7 months (P<0.05), but *before* a short reinforcement programme.

In addition, in the Scottish trial a frequency distribution of examined tooth surfaces scoring plaque index = 0, or 2+ at baseline, after the programme (5 weeks) and before reinforcement (28 weeks) shows that short-term improvements were recorded for both incisors and molars at 5 weeks. After 28 weeks a greater proportion of these improvements had been retained in the molar region (Table 11.2).

Data collected from teachers' questionnaires showed that teachers found the materials to be educationally acceptable (80% to 90%) and pupils to be interested (87%) and comprehending (78%). The data also indicated that over the programme, teachers showed a 50% increase in confidence and enthusiasm increased from 64% to 84%. The impact of teaching style upon the programme was the subject of interest since it helped to elucidate the meaning of clinical outcomes. A dominant style would include directing pupils in their activities, whilst a cooperative style would include giving maximum chance for discussion and pupil ideas.

Using data collected by fieldworkers on standardized schedules and correlating these with plaque and gingival scores, it was possible to discern the importance of teaching style upon improved oral hygiene. Table 11.3 gives a breakdown of dominance, neutral or cooperative styles with measured oral hygiene.

This breakdown may show the importance of style and it was clear from factor analysis that whilst a cooperative style was used with a minority of pupils – and least with the below average ability levels – it has correlated more strongly than other variables (such as ethnicity, sex, or social class) with oral hygiene improvement.[23]

The results of the 'Natural Nashers' trials

Table 11.3 Cross-tabulation of classroom interaction with changes in pupil oral hygiene "Natural Nashers" implementation trials 1980 (%).

	Pupil Ability Level											
	Below average				Average				Above average			
	Oral hygiene				Oral hygiene				Oral hygiene			
	W	S	B	%	W	S	B	%	W	S	B	%
Classroom interaction												
Dominance	53	33	54	51	29	21	28	27	20	22	8	15
Neutral	30	33	15	24	57	52	41	49	57	51	64	59
Cooperation	15	33	29	24	12	25	30	22	22	25	27	25
n =	39	12	44	95	124	51	143	318	121	35	132	288
	x^2	=	4.63		x^2	=	3.39		x^2	=	9.1	
	4df.		N.S.		fdf.		Sig. .01		4df.		Sig. .1	

W = worse; S = same; B = better.

have indicated the feasibility of moving to the next stage, i.e. dissemination. With certain exceptions, this process is in contrast to the familiar pattern of ambitious dental health campaigns where objectives are unspecified, outcomes remain hidden and data collected scant. This pattern may account for the lack of reports in the literature.

Future Developments

In a recently published document, the Health Education Council has included the following objectives for future dental health:

1. To reduce daily frequency of sugar intake among 5 and 14-year-olds.
2. To increase the proportion of 5-year-olds who brush their teeth daily.
3. To increase the proportion of 14-year-olds with a low plaque score.
4. To increase the proportion of 16–20-year-olds with a low plaque score.
5. To increase the proportion of selected handicapped groups who can effectively brush their teeth daily.
6. To increase the proportion of low plaque scores amongst middle-aged (35–50 years) patients with periodontal disease.
7. To increase the proportion of selected elderly groups (65+) with efficient prostheses, and with low plaque scores on standing teeth.

This approach is consistent with the policy of identifying discrete target groups at high risk from dental disease and who have specific needs and characteristics for whom a priority approach is needed that merits specific research and separate motivation programmes. By using such a policy it is not implied that wider structural problems are ignored that contribute to risk – these problems must be tackled as well, but any attempt to do so is at present beyond the power of any existing national agency, separately or together, and must await separate research and Government action. For the present, workers in DHE need to discover structural factors and design their motivation programmes accordingly. That this constrained approach can succeed is demonstrated by the 'Natural Nashers' programme outlined.

Objectives 1, 2 and 3 are covered by the existing work of the Health Education Council Dental Health Study.

Young adults (16–20 years)

The need for a self-care programme arises because of the high risk status of this group. Not only are a very high proportion unemployed, and accident rates high, but many are either embarking on independence or becoming first-time parents. Programmes for this group would aim to be accepted in workplaces, be elective and cater for individual problems. Objectives would include lowered plaque scores on posterior teeth and dietary discrimination.

Middle-age (35–50 years)

Many in this age group will develop periodontal disease, especially if a periodontal epidemic occurs, when dental health workers in practice might expect a large increase in presenting signs and symptoms. Programmes for this group would aim at primary prevention, but also chairside motivation, including elements of treatment (secondary prevention).

Objectives would include reduced plaque levels on posterior teeth, threshold levels of attachment and mobility and evidence of knowledge and positive attitudes.

The disabled and handicapped

Impairment has been defined as physical limitation, whilst disability implies functional restriction and handicap has social and psychological dimensions. Thus loss of a single tooth may be an impairment, but not necessarily a disability or handicap. Loss of a limb may be a disability and a handicap, whilst Downs Syndrome may confer impairment, disability and handicap.

Equally, it follows that impairment may exist without disability or the perception of handicap.

The problem with periodontal disease is that, given cultural and socioeconomic variables, a combination of impairment, disability or handicap may exist. For example, in raising awareness of the disease, a dental health educator may actually *introduce* handicap not previously perceived. But for people already disabled or handicapped by non-dental conditions, periodontal disease will mean additional handicap. As it is, the handicapped (about 1.5 millions in the UK), receive a very small proportion of national resources, and their numbers are likely to increase. The challenge of prevention for this group can no longer be ignored. The objectives of motivation programmes might be:

1. Large and significant reductions of mouth plaque scores in selected groups.
2. Curriculum innovations for use in special schools that combine dental health with educational milestones.

These objectives would demand objective clinical evaluation, but also qualitative and sensitive case studies amongst teachers, health workers and others.

The elderly

The UK population over the age of 65 has increased dramatically this century and now numbers 7.5 million (1981). Already, large numbers live alone in squalor and poverty and without social support. Many are disabled and have multiple health problems for which no immediate solu-

157

tions are available. The whole area of aging and retirement is a major cause for concern, and dental problems form one part of this gloomy picture. There can be no doubt that a functional and aesthetic dentition is as important to an elderly person as any other, and given the poor diet of many elderly people, of particular importance. Falling caries rates may mean a huge increase in the elderly dentate with associated periodontal problems and, here again, a dual approach would be appropriate:

1. Primary prevention aimed at self-care, plaque control and appropriate dietary choice.
2. Chairside programmes of tertiary prevention with treatment and prosthetic input.

Objectives would be framed in terms of plaque reductions, dietary analysis and prosthetic efficiency. Case studies would also be appropriate.

National Strategy for Co-Ordinated Prevention

This review began by drawing attention to the developing concensus in the UK on the need for prevention. Arising from this background, the need for a national strategy for prevention[25] is urgent because treatment services alone will never overcome the social conditions that produce disease. The resources needed for effective prevention of first symptoms would be far too great for the profession alone, even if it could agree on messages and methods! Presumably, it was this that the authors of *Towards Better Dental Health*[55] had in mind when they said: 'a national strategy for dental health would seek to harness and co-ordinate the efforts of all agencies active in the field, commercial as well as professional', adding that, 'health

authorities should finance and evaluate dental health education programmes'.

Such an initiative could transform the present *ad hoc* situation in which agencies feel largely free to pick target groups at will and work in a wastefully competitive atmosphere. In fact, the leading UK commercial and professional agencies have met twice in the last 18 months to exchange information and discuss overall cooperation. At these meetings it was encouraging to find a wide measure of agreement on guiding principles. For example, it was agreed that DHE should be integrated into general health education, directed towards specific target groups, based on agreed and accurate messages and educational principles, and supported by research and evaluation.

If all the major agencies were able to work more closely together, several mutual advantages would be possible and the future for dental health would be improved. Agreement would be needed on broad working principles: consistency of messages and methods; harmony on target groups, desired outcomes and evaluation; longterm integration and compatibility with general health education. Professional agencies could contribute scientific accuracy, enhanced credibility and evaluation skills. The commercial agencies would bring dissemination expertise from marketing and huge advantages in presentation, audiovisual aids and promotion. Each could keep control of separate programmes, but a central coordinating body, perhaps subsidised by a small annual contribution from each, would help to avoid overlap and organise evaluation.

There can be little doubt that industry needs professional legitimation and that the profession needs the experience and resources of industry. The results of real cooperation might be a new public interest in health education and, within 10 years, dental disease might at last be truly under control.

References

1. American Dental Association. Council on dental health and health planning. Changes in the prevalence of dental disease. J. Amer. Dent. Assoc., 1982, 105: 75–79.

2. *Anderson R. J.*
The changes in the dental health of 12-year-old school children in two Somerset schools. A review after 15 years. Brit. Dent. J., 1981, 150: 221.

3. An inquiry into dental education. A report to the Nuffield Foundation. The Nuffield Foundation, 1980, p. 82.

4. *Axelsson P.* and *Lindhe J.*
The effect of a preventive programme on dental plaque, gingivitis and caries in schoolchildren. Results after one and two years. J. Clin. Periodontol., 1974, 1: 126–138.

5. *Axelsson P., Lindhe, J.* and *Wäseby J.*
The effects of various plaque control measures on gingivitis and caries in schoolchildren. Community Dent. Oral Epidemiol., 1976, 4: 232–239.

6. *Axelsson P.* and *Lindhe J.*
Effect of controlled oral hygiene procedures on caries and periodontal disease in adults. J. Clin. Periodontol., 1978, 2: 133–151.

7. *Bingham S., Campbell A.* and *Craft M.*
School meals survey in a Cambridgeshire secondary school. (In press), 1984.

8. British Dental Association. Dental Manpower Requirements to 2020. Report of a Council working party, 1982. pp. 5–6.

9. British Dental Journal. Declining prevalence of dental caries. Editorial, 1982, 153: 4.

10. Child Poverty Action Group. Badge of Poverty, 1982.

11. *Clerehugh V.*
The epidemiology of early periodontal disease in adolescents. The Sir Wilfred Fish Research Prize, 1982. (Unpublished.)

12. *Cochrane A. L.*
Effectiveness and Efficiency: Random Reflections on Health Services. Nuffield Provincial Hospitals Trust, 1972.

13. *Coffield F., Robinson P.* and *Sarsby J.*
A cycle of Deprivation? A Case Study of Four Families. Heinemann Education Books, London, 1980, pp. 157–192.

14. Commission of the European Communities. Final report from the Commission to the Council on the first programme of pilot schemes and studies to combat poverty. Com. (81), 1981, Brussels, pp. 80–85.

15. *Court S. D. M.*
Fit for the Future. Report of the Committee on Child Health Services, HMSO, London, 1976.

16. *Cowell C. R., Saxton C. A., Sheiham A.* and *Wagg B. J.*
Testing the therapeutic measures for controlling chronic gingivitis in man: a suggested protocol. J. Clin. Periodontol., 1975, 2: 231–240.

17. *Cowell C. R.* and *Sheiham A.*
Promoting Dental Health. King Edward's Hospital Fund, London, 1981. pp. 94–103.

18. *Craft M.* and *Croucher R. E.*
The 16–20 study. Dental visiting, knowledge, attitudes and reported behaviour of a national sample of young adults, 16–20 years old. HEC Dental Health Study, University of Cambridge, 1980, pp. 123–130.

19. *Craft M.* and *Croucher R. E.*
The 16–20 study, 1980. Op. cit. pp. 3–7.

20. *Craft M., Croucher R. E.* and *Dickinson J.*
Whole healthy or diseased disabled teeth? Results of pilot studies and controlled feasibility trials. Monograph Number 4. Health Education Council, London, 1981.

21. *Craft M., Croucher R. E.* and *Dickinson J.*
Preventive dental health in adolescents: short and long term pupil response to trials of an integrated curriculum package. Community Dent. Oral Epidemiol., 1981, 9: 201–202.

22. *Craft M., Croucher R. E.* and *Dickinson J.*
Health education in schools: response of biology teachers to a dental health curriculum module. J. Biol. Educ., 1981, 15: 285–288.

23. *Craft M., Croucher R. E.* and *Blinkhorn A.*
Natural Nashers Dental Health Education Programme: results of a trial in Scotland. Brit. Dent. J. 1984, 156: 103–106.

24. *Craft M., Croucher R. E.* and *Dickinson J.*
Teachers as opinion leaders. Dental health education in secondary schools, pp. 499–511. In Health Education and the Media, Leather, D.S., Hastings, G.B. and Davies, J.K. Eds. Pergamon Press, Oxford, 1981.

25. *Craft, M.*
A critical moment for dental health education? Brit. Dent. J., 1982, 153: 214.

26. Department of Education and Science. Numbers of pupils taking school meals. Press Notice, January, 1981; February, 1982.

27. *Doyal L.*
The Political Economy of Health. Pluto Press, 1979, London, pp. 12–13.

28. *Greene J. C.*
Oral hygiene and periodontal disease. Amer. J. Public Health, 1963, 53: 913–922.

29. *Hughes J. T., Rozier R. G.* and *Bawden J. W.*
A survey of periodontal disease in a state population: an emphasis on children. Pediatr. Dent., 1981, 3: Special issue, pp. 114–120.

30. Inequalities in health. Report of a Research Working Group (Sir Douglas Black). Department of Health and Social Security, 1980, London.

31. *Jeffery R.*
Normal rubbish: deviant patients in casualty departments. Sociology of Health and Illness, 1979, 1:1 pp. 99.

32. *Kennedy I.*
Unmasking medicine. The Listener, 1980, London. (November 6th to December 11th.)

33. *Knightley P., Gillie O.* and *Lipsey D.*
The National Health Service: The truth they dared not speak at Brighton. The Sunday Times, 10th October, 1982.

34. *Lennon M.* and *Davies R. M.*
Prevalence and distribution of alveolar bone loss in a population of 15 year old schoolchildren. J. Clin. Periodontol., 1974, 1: 175–182.

35. *Lindhe J.* and *Nyman S.*
The effect of plaque control and gingival pocket elimination on the establishment and maintenance of periodontal health. J. Clin. Periodontol., 1975, 2: 67–79.

36. *Löe H.*
The natural history of periodontal disease in man. J. Periodontology, 1978, 49: 607–620.

37. *Löe H.*
The gingival index, the plaque index and the retention index system. J. Periodontol., 1967, 38: 610–616.

38. *McKeown T.*
The role of medicine: Dream, Mirage or Nemesis? Nuffield Provincial Hospitals Trust, 1976.

39. National Dairy Council. What are Children Eating These Days? 1982.

40. *Naylor M. N.*
The declining prevalence of dental caries. Brit. Dent. J., 1982, 153: 151–152.

41. New Society. Notes: second class fare. 15th April, 1982.

42. Office of Health Economics. Trends in European health spending. Briefing No. 14. 1981. OHE, London.

43. Office of Health Economics. Physical Impairment: Social Handicap, 1977, OHE, London, pp. 3.

44. Prevention and Health: Everybody's business. A reassessment of public and personal health. Department of Health and Social Security, 1976, London.

45. Prevention and health. White Paper. Department of Health and Social Security, 1977, London.

46. Priorities for health and personal social services in England. A consultative document. Department of Health and Social Security, 1976, p. 17., London.

47. *Ramfjord S. P., Knowles J. W., Nissle R. R., Schick R. A.* and *Burgett F. G.*
Longitudinal study of periodontal therapy. J. Periodontol., 1973, 44: 66–67.

48. Royal Commission on the National Health Service. HMSO, 1979, London.

49. Royal Commission on the National Health Service. 1979. op. cit. pp. 339.

50. *Ryan W.*
Blaming the Victim. Vintage Books, 1971, New York.

51. *Sheiham A.*
Dental cleanliness and chronic periodontal disease. Brit. Dent. J., 1970, 129: 413–418.

52. *Steuart G. M.*
Planning and evaluation in health education. Int. J. Health Educ., 1969, 12: No. 2.

53. *Stimson G. V.*
Obeying doctors orders: a view from the other side. Soc. Sci. Med., 1974, 8: 97.

54. *Todd, J. E.* and *Walker A. M.*
Adult Dental Health: England and Wales, Vol. 1. Office of Population Censuses and Surveys, 1980.

55. Towards Better Dental Health – guidelines for the future. The Report of the Dental Strategy Review Group. Department of Health and Social Security, 1981, London, pp. 11–18.

56. *Wade Lord.*
Europe and the British Health Service. Bedford Square Press, 1974, pp. 31.

12. The Primary Health Care Approach: Its Relevance to Oral Health

Aubrey Sheiham

Introduction

The 'Primary Health Care Approach' (PHCA) was formulated at the Alma Ata Conference which was attended by representatives of 134 nations and numerous governmental and nongovernmental organizations. Since then it has become the main health care planning philosophy in both underdeveloped and developed countries and underlies the global strategy of *Health For All By The Year 2000*.[11] Although the dental profession were not officially represented at the Alma Ata Conference, the importance of the PHCA to dentistry is great and this short review will outline its main features and then suggest the relevance of its approach to oral health.

Primary health care is a well-established concept. Confusion exists, however, because it has different meanings in different contexts. In its narrowest sense, primary health care means front-line or first-contact care. Although primary health care is still used in this sense, the concept has broadened to encompass a philosophy that went much further than first-contact services, such as those provided by general medical and dental practitioners. This broader philosophy is expressed in the Declaration of Alma Ata:

'Primary health care is essential health care based on practical scientifically sound and socially acceptable methods and technology, made universally accessible to individuals and families in the community through their full participation and at a cost that the community and country can afford to maintain at every stage of their development in the spirit of self-reliance and self-determination.'

This definition of primary health care was deliberately broader than previous descriptions and was underlined by five principles that distinguished it from earlier narrower concepts. These are: equitable distribution, community involvement, focus on prevention, appropriate technology, and a multisectoral approach. These imply:

1. Health (including dental) services must be more equally accessible, not neglecting rural, isolated groups, and the poor.
2. Active participation by the community in their own health decisions is essential.
3. Preventive and promotive approaches rather than curative services should be the focus of health care.
4. The methods and materials used in the health system should be acceptable and relevant, appropriate technology not being synonomous with primitive or poor technology.
5. Health is only a part of total care (education, shelter, nutrition) and should be improved by involving the agricultural, food manufacturing, economic and employment sectors in planning.

161

This broader philosophy has dominated discussions about primary health care since the 1970s and it is distinguished from the narrower definition by referring to it as the 'Primary Health Care Approach'.[8]

One of the major contributions to the broadening of the concept of health care was the attack on the medical model. The medical model is based on molecular and cellular biology and the germ theory of disease as its basic scientific disciplines.[1] It has become clear that social, psychological, behavioural and economic factors are important aspects of health care. This criticism is particularly relevant to dental services where the medical model and the individualistic mechanistic approach have a strong tendency towards using 'magic bullets' like antibiotics, antiseptics and vaccines to eradicate disease. If medical care is changing because of the shortcomings of the medical model, dentistry should definitely be examining the fundamental tenets upon which dental education, dental services and dental health education messages are based.

What are the other implications of the Primary Health Care Approach (PHCA) for oral, health and dental services? The PHCA lays great emphasis on equitable distribution, community involvement, prevention, appropriate technology and a multisectoral approach.

Equitable Distribution of Dental Care

Primary health care aims at providing the whole population with essential health care.

Dental care should be accessible, which implies the continuing and organized supply of care that is geographically, financially, culturally and functionally within easy reach of the whole community. The care has to be appropriate and adequate in content and in amount to satisfy the essential (dental) health needs of the people, and it has to be provided by methods acceptable to them.[9] Of all health services, dental services are one of the least equitably distributed. The services appear to be designed to meet the needs of the providers rather than those of the public.

A small percentage of the population in countries such as the USA, account for a high percentage of expenditure on dental care; 10% had 75% of all expenditure.[5] Indeed, *House*[3] has stated that barriers to access to dental care are a natural consequence of the capitalist system. In addition to sociopsychological factors, dental fees and patient time create formidable barriers.[3]

Dental services are frequently not integrated into the health services; a pattern of provision which is considered to affect the chances of improving utilization of services.

Attempts should be made to reduce the inequity of dental services by developing a sound dental health manpower system and integrating dental with health services.

Community Participation

Dental care systems have been planned and developed without much community participation. The community have demanded dental services and governments and municipalities have provided traditional dental services.

Community participation in deciding on policies and in planning, implementing and controlling programmes is becoming widely accepted. The PHCA recommends that more participation both by the community and by the health personnel is necessary to harmonize views and activities.

The role of significant members of the

community in setting examples (acting as role models) is important in establishing good oral health practices.[2, 6, 7] Indeed, *Horowitz* and *Frazier*[2] consider that the most powerful educational tool for accomplishing improvements in oral health is a planning process in which community leaders involve themselves in defining problems and identifying and implementing solutions. They suggest the following educational strategies that may interest the community in oral health:

- forming groups of representatives from agencies, civic organizations, trade unions, the womens movement, to examine oral health problems in the community;
- helping consumer groups conduct surveys to identify public perceptions of oral health problems and preferred methods of resolving such problems;
- initiating seminars and workshops to bring oral health problems to the attention of community leaders.

Public decision-makers should be fully informed about comparative benefits and costs of oral health programmes before making policy decisions. The benefits of water fluoridation, the reduction in availability of sugar-containing medicines, baby foods, drinks, food and confections and appropriate dental care services should be carefully explained.

Focus on Prevention

The two major dental diseases, dental caries and periodontal disease, can be effectively prevented by available methods. The dental profession should give more emphasis to prevention and less to curative approaches. The decline in dental caries which is occurring in most EEC countries can be enhanced by concentrating on reducing sugar consumption and limiting dental intervention to a minimum. Popula-

tion strategies to control periodontal disease should be implemented with community participation.

Appropriate Technology

'The word "technology" means an association of methods, techniques and equipment which together with the people using them can contribute significantly to solving a health problem.'[9]

The methods used to treat periodontal disease need to be revised. At the International Workshop held under the auspices of the Committee of Medical and Public Health Research on the efficacy of periodontal treatment,[4] many of the commonly used treatments were considered to be either ineffective or damaging. Nevertheless they continue to be widely used. Methods of controlling the use of ineffective treatments should be explored by dental associations and government bodies.

The types of dental health workers will vary by country and community. Many EEC countries are experiencing a surplus in the number of dentists. They are unlikely to contemplate allowing more appropriate ancillary personnel being trained. The highest priority is the training and employment of dental health educators to work in the community as well as in public and general dental health practices.

A Multi-Sectoral Approach to Improving Oral Health

'An acceptable level of health for all by the year 2000 cannot be achieved by the health sector alone. It can only be attained through national political will and the coordinated efforts of the health sector and relevant activities of other social and economic development sectors'.[11] The control and ultimately the elimination of dental caries is dependent on a multisectoral approach involving the agricultural, food manufacturing, advertising, health education and health care sectors. Whilst the EEC policy is to increase the number of outlets for sugar – sugar being grown with subsidies to the farmers – the downstream efforts of the dental profession to discourage sugar consumption will be seriously undermined. Dental associations should make repeated representations to their governments about the need to limit the production and consumption of refined sugars.

The World Health Organization, The Federation Dentaire Internationale and some national dental organizations are committed to the goal of 'health for all by the year 2000'. The dental goals have been set at a level which is achievable rather than on the absence of disease, disability, discomfort and distress. The adoption of some of the concepts of the Primary Health Care Approach will make a significant impact on oral health for all.

References

1. *Engel G. L.*
   The need for a new medical model: a challenge for biomedicine. Science, 1977, 196: 129–136.

2. *Horowitz A. M.* and *Frazier J. P.*
   Effective public education for achieving oral health. J. Family Community Health, 1980, 3: 91–101.

3. *House D. R.*
   Barriers to access to dental care: an economic examination. J. Amer. Coll. Dent., 1978, 45: 160–169.

4. *Shanley D.* (ed.)
   Efficacy of Treatment Procedures in Periodontics. Quintessence Publ. Co. Chicago, 1980.

5. *Schoen M. H.*
   Dental care delivery in the United States. In International Dental Care Delivery Systems. (Ingle J. I and Blair P. eds.) Ballinger Publ. Co. Cambridge, Mass. 1978, 169–197.

6. *Sheiham A.*
   Current concepts in health education. In Efficacy of Treatment Procedures in Periodontics. (Shanley D. ed) Quintessence Publ., Chicago, 1980.

7. *Sheiham A.*
   Promoting periodontal health – effective programmes of education and promotion. Int. Dent. J., 1983, 33: 182–187.

8. *Walt G.* and *Vaughan P.*
   An Introduction to the Primary Health Care Approach in Developing Countries. Ross Institute Publications, London, 1981, No 13.

9. WHO/UNICEF. Primary Health Care. WHO, Geneva, 1978.

10. WHO. Formulating strategies for Health For All by the Year 2000. WHO, Geneva, 1979.

11. WHO. Global Strategy for Health For All by the Year 2000. WHO, Geneva, 1981.

13. A Dental Preventive Programme for Parents and Their Children, Starting at the Age of 1 Year: Results After 5 Years

Wolfgang Krüger

Introduction

It is generally accepted that the longterm success of dental therapy depends, to a large extent, upon the cooperation of the patients. For this reason, every periodontal treatment is doomed to failure if the patient's oral hygiene is insufficient. However, it is often very difficult to establish and maintain an awareness of the importance of dental hygiene on a longterm basis.[23]

Our main problem in motivating a patient is to change habits and attitudes on a longterm basis. Even if we succeed in making the patient understand the necessity of oral hygiene, there is often a discrepancy between this insight and its persistent realization. The same discrepancy is also apparent in other medical problem areas which have a significant behavioural component, e.g. obesity, smoking, excessive drinking.

Behaviour conducive to health is most easily and effectively acquired during early childhood. Since parents provide an extremely important model for good oral hygiene attitudes and habits in the first years of life, it follows that oral preventive efforts should begin with both parents and their infants.

Additional reasons for starting as early as possible are provided by recent epidemiological evidence. Periodontal disease and dental caries are highly prevalent not only in adults, but in infants, pre-school children, school children, as well as adolescents.[5, 8, 10, 11, 20, 21, 22, 33, 34, 36, 43, 45]

In an investigation of 816 children, 3 to 5 years of age, we observed that only 49.9% of 3-year-olds, 27.2% of 4-year-olds, and 15.1% of 5-year-olds had primary teeth free of dental caries[20, 21] (Fig. 13.1).

Sex-related differences in the results were not significant.

Kindergarten attendance also had no significant influence on the prevalence of dental caries. There was a correlation between social class and caries prevalence in primary teeth; however, even among children of higher social status, more than half had primary teeth affected by dental caries. These results are important for the following reasons:[23]

1. Enough is known about the aetiology of dental caries and periodontal disease for parents to prevent the occurence of both diseases during early childhood.
2. Parental influence in early childhood has a pronounced effect not only on the condition of teeth but also on later nutritional and oral hygiene habits.
3. The condition of the primary teeth is of vital importance to the health of the permanent teeth.

These considerations, along with the findings obtained in examinations of 3-year-olds, were the motivating factors which led to the development of a preventive programme in 1976, integrating correct dental behaviour into the general health

165

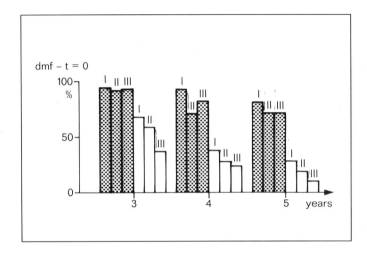

Fig. 13.1 Social Status (I, II, III) and percentage of children with no caries in the prophylaxis group (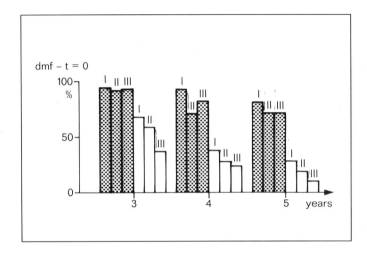) and in the control group (□).[23]

Methods

Main points of programme content

Within the framework of our preventive programme, the following main points have been taken into consideration[17, 23, 24, 39]:

1. Development of confidence between child and dentist by dealing with the child in a friendly and playful manner.
2. Nutritional counselling of parents, pointing out the relationship between sugar consumption and dental caries.
3. Use of toothbrush: Parents are first systematically taught how to properly clean teeth, as well as how to check the efforts of their children. Beginning at the age of 3 years, the children practise in small groups the correct use of the toothbrush.
4. Regular examinations every 6 months.
5. Administration of fluoride-tablets under the control of the parents.
6. Professional cleaning of teeth with a fluoride polishing paste as part of the regular 6-month check-up beginning at age 4 years.
7. Routine treatment of caries and gingivi-

education of children under the age of 3 years. This programme begins with 1-year-olds and incorporates the cooperation of the parents right from its beginning, for only in this way can the parents be informed and motivated to accept the responsibility for the oral hygiene behaviour of their children. The parents must be convinced that their own model behaviour is essential to the dental health education of their children, especially in early childhood.

Our programme was planned on a long-term basis with several preventive appointments per year. This approach is based on our clinical experience and on results of numerous investigations[1, 2, 8, 18, 25, 27] which have shown that the implementation of preventive measures, only once annually, results in practically no improvement. In contrast, a preventive schedule with appointments several times per year, including appropriate comparison measures, shows positive results.[9]

tis as deemed necessary by the regular check-up.

8. Organization of additional prophylactic examinations in cooperation with other clinics within the university (vocal disorders and speech defects; ENT diseases; visual disorders and diseases of the eye).

Programme implementation

While children attending kindergarten or school can be involved in preventive programmes managed by these institutions, younger children can only be reached through their parents. In 1977 in Göttingen all parents with children between the ages of 10 and 18 months were offered the opportunity to participate in our programme. They were informed through pediatricians, radio and the local press. From our own investigations we are aware of the importance of social class factors involved in this procedure.[20] However, considering the pilot nature of our programme, this plays a subordinate role as long as the results are interpreted accordingly.[22, 23, 24]

Since we wanted to develop a concept closely tied to actual practice, two preventive appointments were set up annually for parents and children – each 20 minutes in length during the first 2 years, and 15 minutes thereafter. In addition, at least one evening per year was set aside for a meeting with the parents to pass on basic information and to answer any questions. The individual counselling of parents was the main objective for the first two appointments. They were instructed in the use of the toothbrush, the administration of fluoride-tablets and the implementation of their own correct oral hygiene habits. The children were examined and their oral hygiene behaviours compared. Parents were shown how to determine whether all deposits had really been removed after each brushing. In examining the infant at such an early age it was also our aim to

develop a sense of confidence in the child by gentle and sensitive handling.

Starting at age 3 years, we encouraged that each child began to brush his own teeth properly. We found that practising this in small groups was the best approach. In addition, it was explained to the parents that they were responsible for checking the efficacy of the children's oral hygiene and to repeat the tooth brushing if necessary.

During the check-ups from the age of 4 years on, we cleaned the teeth with a rubbercup and polishing paste containing fluoride.

Study population

Infants and pre-school children

At the first meeting 220 parents were present; at the first preventive appointment 162 children with their parents took part. The mean age of the children was 14.6 months.

Since some families moved in the course of the programme and the social class of several other children could not be definitively established, these children were excluded from the analysis (Table 13.1).

The results were compared to those obtained from examinations of 816 3–5-year-olds.[21, 23] The social class of the participating families was determined according to the criteria of Kleining and Moore,[16] who 'consider the father's occupation as the single best discriminating indicator of the social class' of the whole family. For statistical purposes we combined the social classes into the following groups (Table 13.1; 13.2):

I. Higher middle class = upper and 'middle' middle class
II. Lower middle class
III. Lower class = high and 'low' lower class

Table 13.1 Prophylaxis group: age, number, percentage and social status of children.

Age	Social status							
	I		II		III		Unknown	
	N	%	N	%	N	%	N	%
1	86	53.1	44	27.2	30	18.5	2	1.2
3	58	40.0	37	25.5	33	22.8	17	11.7
4	52	40.9	37	29.1	32	25.2	6	4.7
5	43	38.4	37	33	27	24.1	5	4.5
6–7	43	39.8	37	34.3	27	25.0	1	0.9

Table 13.2 Control group: age, number, percentage and social status of children.

Age	Social status							
	I		II		III		Unknown	
	N	%	N	%	N	%	N	%
3	57	25.9	34	15.5	123	55.9	6	2.7
4	40	16.1	44	17.7	158	63.4	7	2.8
5	58	16.7	64	18.4	221	63.7	4	1.2
6–7	–	–	–	–	–	–	221	100

6 to 7-year-olds

At the beginning of the 1982 school year we performed our 11th check-up within the framework of our programme; 108 children and their parents took part. During the same month the author examined 221 first graders from six different classes in three different schools within Göttingen (S-group) and from four first grade classes in a rural primary school (L-group) (Table 13.3). All children were between 6 and 7 years of age.

For organizational and legal reasons it was not possible to ascertain the social class of all children from this control group.

Examination procedure

Dental caries examination was carried out under standard illumination with mirror and probe on all subjects;[40] the results after 2, 3 and 4 years of the preventive programme were compared to those obtained from the single examination of a group of 3 to 5-year-olds.[23] Since we did not want to overtax the patience and concentration span of the 3 to 5-year-olds, we simply determined the dmft-values and during the preventive programme the plaque index[42] and the gingiva index.[28]

In this study we were, above all, interested in comparing the findings made on children who had taken part in our programme for 5 years (P-group) to those established from the examination of first

Table 13.3 Percentage of children with no caries (DFS + dfs = 0) and mean values ($\bar{x}$) for DFS + dfs in the prophylaxis group (P), urban (S) and rural (L) control group.

| G | N | DFS + dfs = 0 (%) | DFS + dfs ($\bar{x}$) | dispersion[1] | | |
				15%	50% (Median)	85%
P	108	78	0.66	0	0	1
S	130	15	10.78	0	7	21
L	91	11	13.10	2	10	22
S + L	221	14	11.73	1	9	22

[1] dispersion: 15%, 50%, 85% quantile

graders from the city (S-group) and the rural school district (L-group). For this comparison the dfs, dt, ft, dft, DT, FT and DFT values were determined, as were the plaque and gingiva indices.[28, 37, 42]

During our preventive programme we inquired about the living, eating and oral hygiene habits of the families by asking the parents to answer a standardized questionnaire once a year.[23, 24]

Results

Infants and pre-school children

The best parameter in establishing the success of our preventive programme within this age group was that of dental caries prevalence since, even with a lack of oral hygiene, we were seldom able to determine the presence of gingivitis.

In the P-group 93.6% of the children at the age of 3 years were free of caries, whereas only 49.9% of those in the control-group were caries-free; of the 4-year-olds in the P-group, 84.5% were free of caries as opposed to 27.2% in the control group; among 5-year-olds the results were 77.9% versus 15.1% (Fig. 13.1). The mean values ($\bar{x}$) for dmft of 3-year-olds in our P-group was 0.15%, as opposed to

1.77% in the control group; for 4-year-olds, 0.39% versus 2.78% and for 5-year-olds 0.66% versus 3.44% (Fig. 13.2).[23] During our single examination we could find a difference of caries prevalence according to social status,[20] but the verification of the data of our preventive programme according to the Chi-Square-Test did not show any significant differences (Fig. 13.1; 13.2).[23]

Sixty per cent of the 4-year-olds and 53% of the 5-year-olds in the preventive programme received a fluoride tablet every day; the prevalence of dental caries in these children was not significantly different from that in children who did not receive fluoride tablets regularly. In our study a difference in the prevalence of dental caries between these children and those children who did not receive fluoride tablets regularly could not be confirmed. But, since sample size was too small and because of a lack of variation in the frequency of dental caries, a generalization of this finding is questionable.

6 to 7-year-olds

While children, even those with poor oral hygiene, rarely exhibit fully developed gingivitis, we were able to discern and clinically verify detrimental gingival changes in 6 and 7-year-olds. As a result, we used

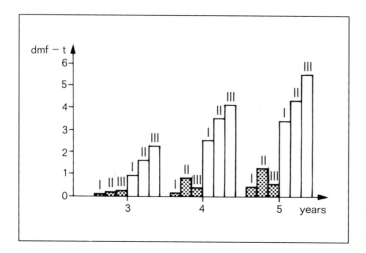

Fig. 13.2 Social Status (I, II, III) and mean values ($\bar{x}$) for dmft of children in the prophylaxis group (▨) and in the control group (☐).[23]

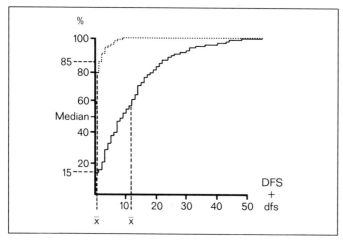

Fig. 13.3 Cumulative frequency in percent of DFS+dfs in the prophylaxis group (P:...) and in the control groups (S+L: —).

caries prevalence, plaque development and gingival changes as parameters to evaluate the success of the programme.

Table 13.3 shows that 78% of the children of our preventive programme (P-group) had neither cavities nor fillings (DFS+dfs=0) in contrast to 15% of the children from the city (S-group) and 11% of the children from the rural area (L-group). The mean values of dfs, as well as the values obtained at 15% quantile, 50% quantile (median) and 85% quantile, clearly show the differences between data obtained from the preventive programme subjects (P) and the control group (S+L).

The cumulative frequency of DFS+dfs is shown in Figure 13.3. Since there were minimal differences between the S- and L-control groups and no additional information could be derived from keeping them separate, the results from these groups were combined into one group (S+L).

Table 13.4 Percentage of children with no decayed primary teeth (dt = 0) and mean values ($\bar{x}$) for dt in the prophylaxis group (P), urban (S) and rural (L) control group.

G	N	dt = 0 (%)	dt ($\bar{x}$)	15%	dispersion[1] 50% (Median)	85%
P	108	86	0.19	0	0	0
S	130	28	3.34	0	3	7
L	91	26	3.8	0	3	8
S + L	221	28	3.53	0	3	7

[1] dispersion: 15%, 50%, 85% quantile

Table 13.5 Percentage of children with no filled primary teeth and mean values ($\bar{x}$) for ft in the prophylaxis group (P), urban (S) and rural (L) control group.

G	N	ft = 0 (%)	ft ($\bar{x}$)	15%	dispersion[1] 50% (Median)	85%
P	108	85	0.42	0	0	0
S	130	62	0.95	0	0	2
L	91	60	1.16	0	0	3
S + L	221	62	1.04	0	0	3

[1] dispersion: 15%, 50%, 85% quantile

Table 13.6 Percentage of children with no decayed and filled primary teeth and mean values ($\bar{x}$) for dft in the prophylaxis group (P), urban (S) and rural (L) control group.

G	N	dft = 0 (%)	dft ($\bar{x}$)	15%	dispersion[1] 50% (Median)	85%
P	108	78	0.61	0	0	1
S	130	22	4.29	0	4	8
L	91	16	4.97	0	5	9
S + L	221	19	4.57	0	4	8

[1] dispersion: 15%, 50%, 85% quantile

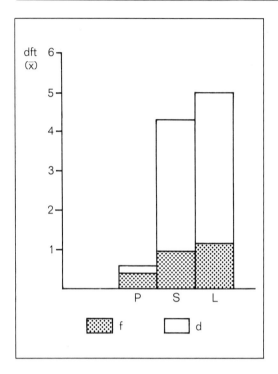

f
d

Fig. 13.4 Mean values (x̄) for decayed and filled primary teeth in the prophylaxis group (P), urban (S) and rural (L) control group.

In Table 13.4, 13.5, 13.6 and in Figure 13.4 and 13.5 the appropiate values for caries (d) and fillings (f) are listed. The differences between the participants and the control groups are clearly visible; while 78% of the children in the preventive group (P) had no teeth affected by caries, this was true of only 19% of the control groups (S+L).

The number of cavities and fillings found in permanent teeth are shown in Table 13.7, 13.8 and 13.9. Additionally, the differences between programme participants (P) and the control groups (S+L) are clearly evident. Of the children in the programme, 99% had healthy permanent teeth as opposed to only 29% of the city control group (S) and 34% of the rural control group (L).

Even though the level of treatment is better in city children (Fig. 13.6; 13.7), the 15%, 50% and 85% quantiles show that differences between the S- and L-groups are not significant (Table 13.7; 13.8; 13.9). For this reason data on the control groups was pooled for calculation of cumulative relative frequency (Fig. 13.6). The values for the plaque and gingiva indices are given in Figures 13.10 and 13.11. A clear difference between children in the programme (P) and children from the control groups (S+L) is evident: 56% of the P-group had no deposits compared to 5% of the S- and 12% of the L-group. No child from the preventive programme was observed with gingivitis, while only 36% of the S-group and 60% of the L-group were not affected by gingivitis. The proportions of children from the S-group with deposits and gingivitis is larger than in the L-group.

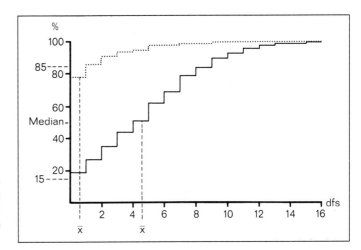

Fig. 13.5 Cumulative frequency in percent of dft in the prophylaxis group (P: . . .) and in the control groups (S + L: —).

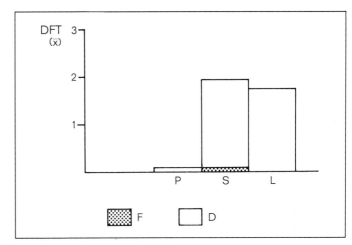

Fig. 13.6 Mean values ($\bar{x}$) for decayed and filled permanent teeth in the prophylaxis group (P), urban (S) and rural (L) control group.

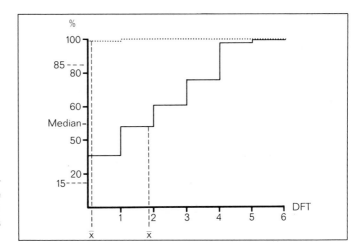

Fig. 13.7 Cumulative frequency in percent of DFT in the prophylaxis group (P: . . .) and in the control groups (S + L: —).

Table 13.7 Percentage of children with no decayed permanent teeth (DT = 0) and mean values ($\bar{x}$) for DT in the prophylaxis group (P), urban (S) and rural (L) control group.

G	N	DT = 0 (%)	DT ($\bar{x}$)	15%	dispersion[1] 50% (Median)	85%
P	108	99	0.01	0	0	0
S	130	29	1.95	0	2	4
L	91	34	1.74	0	1	4
S + L	221	32	1.81	0	2	4

[1] dispersion: 15%, 50%, 85% quantile

Table 13.8 Percentage of children with no filled permanent teeth and mean values ($\bar{x}$) for FT in the prophylaxis group (P), urban (S) and rural (L) control group.

G	N	FT = 0 (%)	FT ($\bar{x}$)	15%	dispersion[1] 50% (Median)	85%
P	108	100	0	0	0	0
S	130	96	0.08	0	0	0
L	91	99	0.01	0	0	0
S + L	221	97	0.05	0	0	0

[1] dispersion: 15%, 50%, 85% quantile

Table 13.9 Percentage of children with no decayed and filled permanent teeth and mean values ($\bar{x}$) for DFT in the prophylaxis group (P), urban (S) and rural (L) control group.

G	N	DFT = 0 (%)	DFT ($\bar{x}$)	15%	dispersion[1] 50% (Median)	85%
P	108	99	0.01	0	0	0
S	130	29	1.95	0	2	4
L	91	33	1.75	0	1	4
S + L	221	31	1.86	0	2	4

[1] dispersion: 15%, 50%, 85% quantile

Table 13.10 Percentage of children with no plaque and mean values ($\bar{x}$) of Plaque-Index (28) in the prophylaxis group (P), urban (S) and rural (L) control group.

G	N	PI = 0 (%)	PI ($\bar{x}$)	15%	dispersion[1] 50% (Median)	85%
P	108	56	0.18	0	0	0.25
S	130	5	1.32	1.00	1.17	2.00
L	91	12	1.15	0.50	1	1.75
S + L	221	8	1.25	1.00	1.17	2.00

[1] dispersion: 15%, 50%, 85% quantile

Table 13.11 Percentage of children with no gingivitis and mean values ($\bar{x}$) of gingiva index (42) in the prophylaxis group (P), urban (S) and rural (L) control group.

G	N	GI = 0 (%)	GI ($\bar{x}$)	15%	dispersion[1] 50% (Median)	85%
P	108	100	0	0	0	0
S	130	36	0.31	0	0.17	0.67
L	91	60	0.39	0	0	1.00
S + L	221	46	0.34	0	0.17	0.75

[1] dispersion: 15%, 50%, 85% quantile

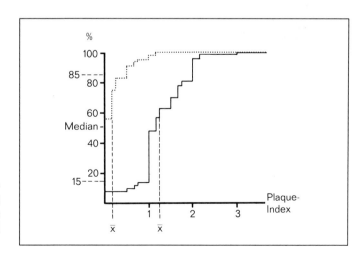

Fig. 13.8 Cumulative frequency in percent of plaque index (28) in the prophylaxis group (P: ...) and in the control groups (S+L: —).

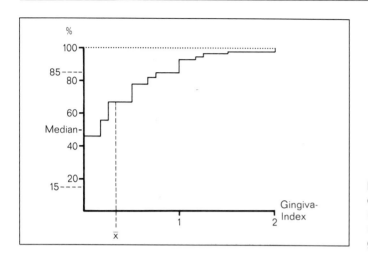

Fig. 13.9 Cumulative frequency in percent of gingiva-index (42) in the prophylaxis group (P: . . .) and in the control groups (S + L: —).

Discussion and Conclusions

The prevalence of dental caries was used to measure the success of our preventive programme in 3 to 5-year-old children. For 6 and 7-year-olds, we used a plaque index[42] and a gingiva index,[28] as well as caries prevalence to evaluate the efficacy of the programme.

One result of our investigation was that we could not confirm a relationship between fluoride intake and prevalence of dental caries. However, a more sophisticated research design is needed to satisfactorily investigate this important question and this finding cannot therefore be generalized.

We found clear differences between programme participants and control groups in all age groups with respect to dental caries development. The results we obtained in terms of age-dependent caries development are in agreement with results obtained by other investigators.[4, 5, 6, 11, 30, 41, 43, 44, 46, 48] The children in the preventive programme exhibited few differences between age groups. Whereas 50% of the children in our control group developed caries after one year, this was true of only

10% of an age group in our preventive programme.

In the group of 6 to 7-year-olds there were also considerable differences between preventive programme participants and the control group, not only for the primary teeth (dft) but even for the few permanent teeth (DFT). The difference between P-, S- and L-groups are also striking in terms of plaque and gingiva indices. The insufficiency of oral hygiene in the control groups is apparent in both milk-teeth and permanent teeth. This pattern was previously noted by *Jacobs*[14] in 1936, who found only 2.5% of the 6-year-olds in Göttingen to be free of dental caries. Numerous other investigators have also documented the poor conditions of teeth in first graders.[3, 5, 10, 12, 15, 26, 33, 43, 44, 45, 47]

A main problem of interpreting the results of our investigation is the selection bias which develops as a result of the voluntary nature of our preventive programme. The fact that our experimental group is strongly skewed towards the upper social classes might lead critics to the conclusion that our programme did not show much positive effects since the prevalence of dental caries in the upper social classes is lower anyway. But since our one-time examination showed that even in the upper social classes 27.2% of the 5-year-olds were unaffected by dental caries as opposed 80.4% in our prophylaxis group,[23] we feel that our preventive programme was quite effective. The fact that our experimental group did not exhibit a significant relationship between prevalence of dental caries and social class also shows that social class variables may be of less importance for the effectiveness of preventive dental health measures than previous research indicate.[3, 11, 13, 47] We rather feel that motivational factors which have been widely neglected in dental research until recently may have a great influence on the good results of our prophylaxis group.

The results on 6 and 7-year-olds in urban area and those in rural area differ only slightly and should be re-examined in further studies. Nearly half of the 6 and 7-year-olds exhibited clinically confirmed gingivitis. Similar results were obtained by other investigators for 5 and 6-year-olds.[7, 8, 29, 30, 32, 36] Gingivitis was not detected in children participating in the preventive programme. A similar difference between programme and control groups was found with the respect to plaque indices. We attribute these results to the fact that the parents were incorporated into our programme.

Parents and children are thereby influenced right from the start, so dental caries and periodontal disease can be largely prevented. A positive attitude toward oral hygiene establishes the optimal basis for healthy permanent teeth and the realization of life-long dental prevention.

Our results support *Kriesberg* and *Treiman*[19, 23] in their conclusions from studies on adolescents that there are three determining factors involved in establishing preventive health behaviour:

1. Knowledge and attitude of the parents.
2. Attitude of the dentist.
3. Age at first dental visit.

The common failure of attempts to influence oral hygiene habits of children, adolescents and adults[38] can generally be attributed to two interrelated factors:

1. Preventive measures are implemented too late, when attitudes and behaviours with respect to oral hygiene are already established.
2. The significant role of the parents in early childhood is not taken into consideration.

Ulvestad and *Gilinsky*[49] have also attributed the reduction of caries prevalence in 3-year-olds to the fact that the parents were informed about preventive measures. *Schwarz* and *Hansen*[41] report that by 1987 all children in Denmark between the ages of 1 year and 16 years will be under dental supervision; the individual communities will be responsible for the organization and implementation of this programme. Prompted by the results of our studies, we have met with representatives of health insurance companies, the local dental association, and the Public Health Department to plan a cooperative comprehensive preventive programme. The programme will start with the eruption of the first deciduous tooth, and it will be implemented in 1983[24.1, 48]: Parents receive a 'check-up book' from their health insurance company for each child from one year of age on. This book instructs the parents when to bring their children to the dentist for regular 6 month examinations. Each dentist also receives detailed instructions concerning preventive procedures, thereby assuring the same controls as in our preventive programme.

Acknowledgements

I am greatly appreciative of the qualified guidance given to me by Mrs *R. Turgut*, Dipl.-Psych., and Mr *P. Keßler*, Dipl. Math., in helping with the calculation and interpretation of the results of this study.
I would also like to thank Mr *D. Starr*, M. A., Lecturer, and Ms *M. Diermayer*, B. S., Cand. med., for their assistance in translating this manuscript into English.

References

1. *Axelsson P.* and *Lindhe J.*
   The effect of a preventive programme on dental plaque, gingivitis and caries in schoolchildren. Results after one and two years. J. Clin. Periodontol., 1974, 1: 126–138.

2. *Axelsson P.* and *Lindhe J.*
   Effects of controlled oral hygiene procedures on caries and periodontitis disease in adults. J. Clin. Periodontol., 1978, 1: 133–151.

3. *Borggrefe R.*
   Gebiß- und Parodontalbefunde in ihrer Abhängigkeit zur Mundhygiene. Med. Diss., Bonn, 1973.

4. *Druszt P., Banoczy I., Esztary I., Hadas E., Marosi I., Newes I.* and *Albrecht M.*
   Caries prevalence of pre-schoolchildren in Baja, Hungary in 1955 and 1975. Community Dent. Oral Epidemiol., 1977, 5: 136–139.

5. *Cahen J. P.*
   Der Kariesbefall des Milchgebisses bei 4- bis 6-jährigen Kindern in Basel 1962. Med. Diss., Basel, 1962.

6. *Cleaton-Jones P., Richardson B. D., McInnes P. M.* and *Fatty L. P.*
   Dental caries in South African white children aged 1–5 years. Community Dent. Oral Epidemiol., 1978, 6: 78–81.

7. *Curilovic Z.*
   Gingivitis bei Züricher Vorschulkindern. Schweiz. Monatsschr. Zahnheilkd., 1975, 85: 1105–1111.

8. *Curilovic Z., Mazor Z.* and *Berchthold H.*
   Gingivitis in Zürich school children. A reexamination after 20 years. Schweiz. Monatsschr. Zahnheilkd., 1977, 87: 801–808.

9. *Curilovic Z.* and *Meier Ch.*
   Zur parodontalen Prophylaxe und Therapie in der Schweiz. Schweiz. Monatsschr. Zahnheilk., 1980, 90: 79–84.

10. *Gülzow H.-J.*
    Die Karies im Milchgebiß. Dtsch. Zahnärztl. Z., 1968, 12: 1204–1207.

11. *Gülzow H-J., Gerritzen Th.* and *Ritter H.-J.*
    Milchzahnkaries bei Großstadtkindern. Dtsch. Zahnärztl. Z., 1980, 35: 297–300.

12. *Hafen J-P.*
    Statistische Untersuchung über den Zustand des Milchgebisses beim 5- bis 6jährigen Kind. Med. Diss., Zürich, 1955.

13. *Hausen H., Milen A., Heinonen O. P.* and *Paunio I.*
    Caries in primary dentition and social class in high and low fluoride areas. Community Dent. Oral Epidemiol., 1982, 10: 33–36.

14. *Jacobs C.*
    Über die Karieshäufigkeit mit besonderer Berücksichtigung der Milchzahnkaries einerseits, der kariösen Prozesse andererseits. Med. Diss., Göttingen, 1936.

15. *Kahre K.*
    Über den Zustand des Milchgebisses bei vorschulpflichtigen Kindern in Spandau. Med. Diss., Berlin, 1932.

16. *Kleining G.* and *Moore H.*
    Soziale Selbsteinstufung (SSE). Köln Z. Soziol. Sozialpsychol., 1968, 20: 502–552.

17. *Koch A.*
    Die Auswirkungen zahnmedizinischer Prophylaxe auf den Kariesbefall bei Vorschulkindern. Med. Diss., Göttingen, 1984 (in press).

18. *König K.*
    Der Zahnarzt als Gesundheitserzieher. Zahnärztl. Mitt., 1977, 5: 271–273.

19. *Kriesberg L.* and *Treiman B. R.*
    Preventive utilization of dentists' services among teenagers. J. Amer. Coll. Dent., 1962, 29: 28–32.

20. *Krüger W., Mausberg R.* and *Kozielski R. M.*
    Kariesfrequenz, Kariesbefall und soziale Milieubedingungen bei Kindern im Vorschulalter. Dtsch. Zahnärztl. Z., 1978, 33: 164–166.

21. *Krüger W., Mausberg R.* and *Kubein D.*
    Kariesbefall und Behandlungsnotwendigkeit bei Kindern im Vorschulalter. Dtsch. Zahnärztl. Z., 1979, 35: 110–112.

22. *Krüger W., Rutschmann A.* and *Mausberg R.*
    Karies- und Gingivitis-Prophylaxe bei Vorschulkindern – unser Langzeitprogramm. Dtsch. Zahnärztl. Z., 1980, 35: 1061–1064.

23. *Krüger W., Koch A.* and *Rutschmann A.*
    Gingivitis- und Kariesprophylaxe für Kinder vom

ersten bis zum fünften Lebensjahr: Das Langzeit-Prophylaxe-Programm Göttingen (1977–1981). Dtsch. zahnärztl. Z., 1982, 37: 557–564.

24. *Krüger W.*
Karies- und Gingivitis-Prophylaxe bei Kleinkindern. Hüthig, Heidelberg, 1983.

24. *Krüger W.*
Kariesbefall, Mundhygiene und Gingivitis bei Schulanfängern. Kariesprophylaxe, 1984: 115–120.

24.1 *Krüger W., Turgut R.* and *Schwibbe G.*
Aktion „Gesunde Zähne vom 1. Milchzahn an": Zur Realisierung von Prophylaxe-Maßnahmen in der zahnärztlichen Praxis. Oralprophylaxe 1984 (in press).

25. *Lange D.*
Hygienekontrolle bei instruierten und motivierten Patienten. In Prophylaxe. (Peters S., ed.) Quintessenz, Berlin, 1978.

26. *Lehm F.*
Konservierende Behandlung des Milchgebisses, Schulzahnpflege in Göttingen von Ostern 1912 bis Ostern 1921. Med. Diss., Göttingen, 1921.

27. *Lightner L. M., O'Leary T. O., Drake R. B., Crump P. B.* and *Allen M. R.*
Preventive periodontic treatment procedures: Results over 46 months. J. Periodontol., 1971, 42: 555–561.

28. *Löe H.* and *Silness J.*
Periodontal disease in pregnancy. I. Prevalence and severity. Acta Odont. Schand., 1963, 21: 533–551.

29. *Massler M., Cohen A.* and *Schour I.*
Epidemiology of gingivitis in children. J. Amer. Dent. Assoc., 1952, 45: 319–324.

30. *Møller P.*
Oral health survey of preschool children in Iceland. Acta Odont. Scand., 1963, 21: 47–97.

31. *Papperitz K.*
Kariesstatistische Untersuchungen im Jahre 1955 an 1000 Vorschulkindern mit reinem Milchgebiß. Med. Diss., Leipzig, 1957.

32. *Parfitt G. J.*
A five-year longitudinal study of the gingival conditions of a group of children in England. J. Periodontol., 1957, 28: 26–30.

33. *Patz J.* and *Gülzow H.-J.*
Epidemiologie der Zahnkaries. Münch. Med. Wochenschr., 1977, 119: 381–386.

34. *Patz J.* and *Naujoks R.*
Morbidität und Versorgung der Zähne in der

Bevölkerung der Bundesrepublik Deutschland. Dtsch. Zahnärztl. Z., 1980, 35: 259–264.

35. *Plasschaert A. J. M., König K. G.* and *Vogels A. L. M.*
Onderzoek naar de gebitstoestand van kinderen in Nordoost Friesland. Ned. Tijdschr. Tandheelkd., 1974, 81: 342–346.

36. *Poulsen S.* and *Møller I. J.*
The prevalence of dental caries, plaque and gingivitis in 3-year-old Danish children. Scand. J. Dent. Res., 1972, 80: 94–103.

37. Ramfjord S. P.
Indices for prevalence and incidence of periodontal disease. J. Periodontol., 1959, 30: 51–59.

38. *Rayner J. I.* and *Cohen L. K.*
School dental health education. In Social Sciences and Dentistry: A Critical Bibliography. (Richard N. D. and Cohen L. K. eds.) The Hague, Netherlands, A. Sijhoff Publishers, 1971.

39. *Rutschmann A.*
Die Auswirkungen zahnmedizinischer Prophylaxe auf den Kariesbefall bei Kleinkindern. Med. Diss., Göttingen, 1981.

40. *Sauerwein E.*
Kariologie. Thieme, Stutgart, 1974.

41. *Schwarz E.* and *Hansen E.*
Caries experience of Danish children evaluated by the Child Dental Health recording system. Community Dent. Oral Epidemiol., 1979, 7: 107–114.

42. *Silness J.* and *Löe H.*
Periodontal disease in pregnancy. II. Correlation between oral hygiene and periodontal condition. Acta Odont. Scand., 1964, 22: 121–135.

43. *Sittig M.*
Kariesbefall, Mundhygiene und Süßigkeitenkonsum bei 3- bis 10jährigen Aachener Kindern. Med. Diss., Bonn, 1972.

44. *Spiller K.*
Anstieg des Milchzahnkariesbefalls. Zahnärztl. Mitt., 1966, 56: 792–793.

45. *Steinert U.*
Der Kariesbefall der 3- bis 6jährigen in Bonner Kindergärten. Med. Diss., Bonn, 1971.

46. *Sutcliffe P.*
Caries experience and oral cleanliness of 3- and 4-year-old children from deprived and non deprived areas in Edinburgh, Scotland. Community Dent. Oral Epidemiol., 1977, 5: 213–219.

47. *Thelen H.*
Zahn- und Parodontalverhältnisse bei 3- bis

9jährigen Kindern im Rhein-Hunsrück-Kreis. Med. Diss., Bonn, 1981.

48. *Turgut R., Schwibbe G.* and *Krüger W.:*
Aktion „Gesunde Zähne vom 1. Milchzahn an": Die Rolle der Eltern bei der Gesundheitserziehung. Oralprophylaxe 1984 (in press)

49. *Ulvestad H.* and *Gilinsky A.*
Effect on caries prevalence in 3-year-old children of a preventive program given at child health centre. Swed. Dent. J., 1977, 1: 159–162.

14. Implementation of Preventive Periodontal Programmes at the Community Level

Taco Pilot

Introduction

We know enough of the aetiology, pathogenesis and progress of periodontal disease[13] – at least from a theoretical point of view – to be able to control the disease. It is possible to prevent the disease to a large extent, to apply effective treatment and to prevent further sequelae. The fundamental and basic segments of research have brought forward enough evidence to present a rationale for prevention and treatment of periodontal disease. Successful application of this knowledge has also been demonstrated in numerous scientific articles with case presentations and results of experimental clinical trials. Furthermore, in addition to the experiments discussed in the *EEC Workshop on the Efficacy of Periodontal Treatment Procedures* in Dublin in December 1979, a number of reports have been published worldwide.

More insight has also been provided on the results of periodontal treatment with positive aspects for a more preventive approach of the periodontal problem. There is more optimism on the prognosis of the conservative, nonsurgical methods of treatment.[7, 51, 52, 55, 59] A few, but encouraging reports on periodontal programmes with prevention oriented goals have been published (see p. 186–188). Thus, it is possible to be more optimistic about the feasibility of disease controlling programmes for adults. Perhaps it is also time for a redefinition of the periodontal problem in Europe that leaves less room for pessimism.[47, 68]

Nevertheless, at least one main problem remains, i.e. the implementation of what is known from research into the widespread use at the community level. Periodontal disease continues to represent a major dental health problem in Europe, resulting in much suffering and vast expenditures of public and private money, even though the disease is largely preventable. Periodontal (dental) health in Europe is not in a bad state because of lack of progress in science, technology or skill, nor because of lack of funds – even today in an era of declining economical wealth – but rather because there is such a wide gap between what is scientifically known about the control of disease and what is implemented and practised by dental professionals, health care organisations and the public at large. Apparently there are barriers on the road: the translation of results from research into practical application in society appears to be a difficult task.

The problem of effective use of proven preventive measures by the profession and the general public is an extremely complex one.[17, 19, 24, 25, 26, 39, 58, 62, 63, 65, 66, 73, 74] The problem encompasses numerous decision-making processes involving individuals as well as policy-making bodies, and individual dental health workers as well as professional organisations. Such social-political processes determine the extent to which effective preventive measures are considered, adopted and maintained at the community level. However, research on adoption of effective technologies to prevent oral diseases has been limited.

What are the barriers to the promotion of periodontal (oral) health in Europe? Which factors govern the implementation of preventive periodontal programmes at the community level? It is possible to look at this topic from many different angles, but the most critical part of any health care programme is planning. Thus, it was chosen to look at the implementation problem from the perspective of planning dental health care using WHO documents as baseline.[81, 82, 83, 84, 85, 86, 87, 88]

A number of conditions should be fulfilled from a planning point of view in order to obtain successful implementation of a preventive periodontal programme at the community level. These requirements can be arranged in several, closely related and partly overlapping areas: The preventive periodontal programme should

- be directed to a recognized and commonly accepted major public health problem;
- be based on a sound scientific rationale;
- have clearly defined, time related, measurable goals;
- be acceptable to the 'client' at the community level;
- be relevant and acceptable at the professional level;
- include an evaluation and feedback system.

Requirements for Successful Implementation; a Critical Evaluation

The programme should be directed to a recognized and commonly accepted major public health problem. One might ask: 'Recognized and accepted by whom?

There are at least three separate entities who should recognize and accept periodontal disease as a major public health problem.

Firstly, from a scientific point of view, a health problem is considered an important problem to the community when the prevalence is high and/or the consequences are serious, with emphasis placed on the latter. Consequences are then expressed as impacts on the quality of life and in terms of suffering, chances of disability, or even death. Furthermore, the amounts of manpower/financial resources the problem absorps, both directly in cost of care services and indirectly in loss of working hours, might also be included. Periodontal disease is one of the most widespread diseases in the world. It is the most common cause of loss of teeth in many developing countries. One might also accept statements concerning a high prevalence of periodontal disease in most industrialized countries, including the EEC countries. In these countries, it is also said to be the cause of tooth loss and edentulousness among many persons over 40 years of age, but conclusive evidence for this specific statement is still lacking.

Secondly, the condition should be an important health problem as perceived by the individual and the community, including community leaders, health policy decision-makers and government agencies, and ultimately political decision-makers.

There certainly is a discrepancy between the prevalence of the disease and the need for treatment, as indicated by professionals on the one hand, and the awareness of those people (potentially) affected on the other. This discrepancy will be more striking when awareness has to be converted in politically expressed demand for treatment and preventive procedures. It all comes down to the significance of periodontal disease in society and the concept of disease and illness as explained by *Ainamo*.[1] According to *Waerhaug*,[80] the loss of a front tooth is no longer considered a noble trademark of a labourer, but rather a social disaster. It is also fashionable now to look young, healthy and successful.[1] But the value of a healthy natural dentition and its impact on the quality of life is certainly not a frequent topic of conversation in European family life.

The acceptance of the problem is especially crucial when *preventive* programmes are under discussion. It might be that governments in Europe and elsewhere would like to see a shift away from therapeutic/curative services towards more prevention.[3, 4, 18, 57] Nevertheless, political decision-makers do not like to go against the immediate interest of their voters, who are far less prevention oriented. One wonders where and by whom in society periodontal disease is accepted as a major public health problem?

Thirdly, there is the role of the dental profession and, indirectly, the role of dental educators. Most students choose dentistry because they like a technical job. Most teachers at universities and dental schools reinforce such a set of values and attitudes because it is part of their own concept. This, together with the historical avenue of dental education, provides a barrier to the translation of results of research into the curriculum for the future dental practitioner. So the level of awareness amongst the profession about periodontal disease as a major public health problem might indeed be low. Whenever the problem might have been recognized formally by, for example national organisations of dentists, it is far from being accepted as a major problem which should be attacked by every dentist. What is meant here is the attitude of many a dentist who tries to 'export' the problem: 'They should take care of it', 'they' meaning 'anybody else except me'.

A positive trend might be that the simple market mechanism of lower caries incidence will force dentists to pick up the periodontal business.[3, 4] It is still to be seen, though, whether that helps the implementation of *prevention* oriented periodontal programmes at the community level.

The programme should be based on a sound scientific rationale

We know enough about cause, aetiology and pathogenesis of periodontal disease to establish the scientific basis for prevention and treatment. However, the available evidence is not sufficient for application on a mass scale. There are some gaps in our knowledge and attention has to be paid to at least 5 questions:

1. Do we know enough of the progress of the disease and is it possible to identify high risk groups?
2. Is it justified to carry out screening procedures at the population level?
3. Are there accurate estimates of periodontal treatment needs?
4. Is it possible to formulate adequate goals for a preventive periodontal programme?
5. Are there reports of successful prevention oriented periodontal programmes under real life conditions?

Progress of the disease. Identifying high risk groups

In recent years, some studies have been published on the progress of periodontal disease. The Oslo – Shri Lanka studies[5] on the natural history of periodontal disease (already discussed in the EEC Workshop in Dublin) have brought additional data. Also data of studies by *Selikowitz et al.*[70] were published.

There is growing consensus that periodontal disease does not automatically progress from early gingivitis, with a gradual loss of attachment into the terminal stages of periodontitis for all persons at the same speed. The close relationship that has been demonstrated in large popu-

183

lation groups, over years and throughout the world, between the amounts of bacterial plaque and prevalence and severity of periodontal disease is not questioned at all. But, more evidence suggests that it might be possible in the near future to identify: (1) persons who are more susceptible to progressing periodontal disease than others, (2) periods in one's life where outbursts in disease activity can be recognized in contrast to periods of relative quiesence, and (3) sites in the oral cavity with more risk of progressing loss of attachment. In short, high-risk groups, high-risk periods and high-risk sites!

Prognostic indicators for disease activity of the past were redness, and as signs of gingivitis swelling of the gingiva and bleeding gums. Pocket depths and the rate of loss of periodontal attachment were registered on the assumption that these are predictors of ultimate tooth loss. But the consensus today is that the mere presence of gingivitis or a pocket does not adequately predict progressing loss of attachment. New indicators have been suggested, based on bacteriological sampling/identification,[53, 64, 75] and the clinical sign of bleeding on probing is now incorporated in the new index of treatment need.[2] However, much more research has to be done before practical tools and methods for identifying *high-risk* episodes, or *high-risk* persons are available. There is a strong need for research on prognostic indicators.

The high-risk concept is a positive trend because, by proposing high risk for a small part of the population, one (implicitely) assumes that in the remaining large part of the population the progress of disease will be rather slow. This assumption changes the fatalistic description of the enormous, overwhelming and never to cope with problem in populations, so often heard in the past, to the concept that periodontal disease is a still widespread and difficult, but nevertheless manageable disease.

Requirements for screening

The requirements for screening for periodontal disease have been summarized and discussed extensively by *Sheiham*:[72]

'The prime objective of screening is to detect disease at an earlier stage than would normally occur with people presenting with the disease, on the assumption that earlier treatment would alter the natural history of the disease in a significant proportion. However, before a screening survey is done a number of conditions should be fulfilled. The disease should be an important health problem; there should be effective and acceptable treatment available for those with the disease; the natural history of the disease should be adequately understood and there should be an agreed policy on whom to treat.

Periodontal disease does not fulfil many of the requirements for a disease suitable for population screening. There is no reliable evidence that earlier detection alters the natural history of the disease or the survival and function of the teeth. Neither is there sufficient information on the importance of clinical signs of periodontal disease. We do not know whether screening tests are able to detect periodontal disease which is likely to have an important impact on periodontal health. For example, is bleeding an important sign of destructive periodontal disease?'

At present it seems that although some progress has been made, the conclusion again must be made that *population screening* for periodontal disease is not justified.

Estimates of treatment needs

The above gaps in our knowledge on periodontal disease cast severe doubts on the accuracy of estimates of periodontal treatment needs in populations. There is a growing body of knowledge and data on prevalence, incidence and severity of periodontal disease in the European countries, although the coverage of data is quite uneven. Data on gingivitis, periodontitis, prevalence of pockets and attachment loss are available. However, data of this nature cover only part of the problem. We still do not know enough on the progression of the disease and how that affects loss of function related to the overall goal 'a functioning natural dentition for life'. The old question about causes of tooth loss is not yet answered. To be specific: 'What percentage of extractions is carried out because of periodontal disease in terminal stages?' A redefinition of the periodontal problem in Europe seems appropriate.

Goals for a preventive programme

At the *EEC Workshop on the Efficacy of Periodontal Treatment* in Dublin the available publications on longterm prospective studies on periodontal treatment were summarized.[63] Effective treatment programmes were identified, decisive factors in success were discussed and an attempt was made to indicate adequate levels of plaque control. In conclusion it was stated:

'There is strong scientific evidence that plaque control is the only essential factor in the prevention and treatment of periodontal disease. The current status of periodontology permits the conclusion that periodontal disease can be prevented and periodontal breakdown can be arrested in individuals and in large groups of the population only when an adequate oral hygiene regime is instituted.

'In order to define objectives in plaque control, realistic targets in periodontal health care may be suggested as:

(a) a level of plaque in quantitiy and quality that is compatible with contained gingivitis, that is gingivitis which does not progress into destructive periodontitis;

(b) a level of plaque which leads to a rate of progress of periodontal disease which will not lead to unacceptable gingival recession;

(c) a level of plaque which leads to a rate of progress of periodontal destruction which is compatible with keeping the natural functioning dentition for the life time of the individual.'

The last target is certainly the most important and the remaining question is: 'How much (and what kind of) plaque is tolerable or compatible with a healthy natural functioning dentition for life?'

Thus, it continues to be difficult to formulate adequate goals for a preventive periodontal programme. Furthermore, do we agree on the definition of a functioning dentition? *Käyser*[48] has published some innovative concepts. There might emerge more optimism and less need for extensive restorative/prosthetic care.[48, 61]

Demonstrations of successful prevention oriented programmes

Since the Dublin Workshop, more reports have become available. In studying these, we should keep in mind the difference between an experimental clinical trial and community clinical trial. According to *O'Mullane*[56] 'a clear distinction must be drawn between an experimental clinical trial carried out under ideal conditions and a community clinical trial carried out under real-life conditions. Because of the artificial nature of an experimental trial there are strict limitations placed on its objectives and the inferences that can be drawn from its results. Before a preventive or therapeutic procedure is adopted for use on a public health basis, it must undergo a set sequence of test procedures. Following encouraging results from *in vitro,* laboratory and animal studies a controlled clinical trial is arranged. According to an ideal sequence, if the procedure is found to be effective in a number of independently conducted clinical trials, then a test under real life or field conditions is considered.' In addition, *Lennon*[50] wrote 'an experimental clinical trial to measure effectiveness under the most favorable conditions and a community clinical trial to evaluate cost-effectiveness and acceptability under real life conditions'.

Clinical trials on programmes with prevention oriented goals for adolescents and adults have been performed in Europe in the last couple of years. These are mostly straightforward experimental clinical trials. Only a few have some characteristics of a *community* clinical trial. Attention should be paid to the trials.

1. *Hugoson et al.* in Jönköping, Sweden.[40, 41, 42, 43, 44, 45, 46, 47] Starting in 1973, a dental health care programme was gradually built up for children and adolescents. A continuous training programme was introduced for all dental care personnel.[42] A basic preventive programme was given to all children and adolescents, irrespective of need, and was intended to reduce disease activity in general. Furthermore, there was a supplementary programme intended for individuals who, in spite of the basic programme, continued to exhibit high disease activity.[44]

Reports on the results of the care programme were based on data of 80 individuals, aged 15 years at the time of the first registration and aged 20 years when re-examined in 1978.[45] Plaque, calculus, gingival status, pockets and level of alveolar bone were recorded clinically and radiographically. The prevalence of plaque and gingivitis decreased for buccal and lingual surfaces, but increased approximately. Altogether, 75 tooth surfaces with pocketing were diagnosed in 1973 against 21 in 1978. The level of alveolar bone did not show any differences. The percentage of persons with calculus decreased. The prevalence and incidence during a

5 year period of destructive periodontitis seemed to be rather low. The authors concluded that in spite of the many proximal areas with gingivitis, very few 20-year-olds showed signs of marginal bone loss, which indicates that gingivitis does not necessarily lead to destructive periodontitis in young people. Additional data on the same project, indicating improved periodontal health, have been published in several articles.[41, 46] In the preventive programme initiated, no special emphasis was placed on introducing measures for interproximal cleaning. The result was a demonstration that tooth brushing is not enough to bring about proximal cleaning. The authors believe that, provided due focus is placed on procedures adapted to the need of adults, there is every reason to hope that a corresponding beneficial effect on dental health will also be achieved in the adult population.

In relation to the experimental care programme, epidemiological studies were also carried out,[40, 43, 47] indicating high percentages of gingivitis for the population, but strikingly few cases of severe destructive periodontitis.

2. *Söderholm et al.* in Malmö, Sweden.[11, 12, 31, 77, 78, 79] Dental health was studied in a longitudinal investigation of several hundred blue and white-collar workers at a shipyard in Malmö.[77] Data of earlier periods were also available as controls.[11] The patients received an initial treatment consisting of prophylactic and restorative treatment in 1974 and thereafter continuing preventive care every 3rd month. Each instance of preventive care was performed by specially trained auxiliaries. Discussions on the cost analysis were also made.[12, 77] No differences could be observed between the results of five consecutive 30 minute visits, compared to two 60 minute visits. In both groups, the presence of plaque, gingival bleeding and periodon-

tal pockets were significantly reduced.[78] Another study indicated that three consecutive 30 minute appointments is as effective in instructions as three 15 minute appointments, despite the fact that approximately half of the individuals were immigrants and verbal communication was somewhat difficult.[79] The authors indicate that comprehensive (time-consuming) plaque control programmes may not be necessary and may not increase the effect of basic plaque control instruction.

3. *Hetland, Midtun* and *Kristoffersen* in Sandnes, Norway.[36, 37, 38, 49] The study was undertaken in order to test the effect of hygiene instructions given by specially trained chairside assistants and to test the value of professional prophylaxis prior to instructions. Chairside assistants received an intensive course of 40 hours duration to motivate and instruct patients in oral hygiene methods utilizing a prescribed three-visit programme totalling 1½ hours. Seventy one employees of an industrial firm were divided into three groups, receiving respectively: (a) prophylaxis only, (b) instructions only and (c) prophylaxis before instructions. Participants were examined after 4, 12 and 24 weeks with respect to DMF-T, Gingival Index and bleeding on probing, Retention Index, plaque surfaces and periodontal pockets of 4 mm of depth or more.

Significant improvement was observed in group (b) and (c) for plaque (reduction approximately 70%), gingivitis and pocket depths. As the effects of instructions were retained after 6 months, it was concluded that the use of this type of personnel is highly effective and expedient and that the presented model can be useful in preventive dental health work.

The project was well-accepted both by the employees and the company management and possibilities for a permanent arrangement were discussed. Potential consumers (the employees) were especially interested in two parts of the proposed model: (a) by using a preventive model one will, in a less time-consuming and cheaper way, be able to give the offer to all the employees; (b) those who take care of their teeth and go regularly to the dentist will not have the feeling that they are paying for those who do not take the same care.

4. *Hamp et al* in Linköping, Sweden.[10, 20, 32, 33, 34] The effect of a dental prophylactic programme based on systematic plaque control was tested during a 3-year period on more than 100 youths aged 16–19 years.[33] This study was the follow-up of a caries and gingivitis prophylactic field experiment on 1100 schoolchildren aged 7–16 years reported earlier.[32] The study showed that it is possible during a 3-year period to effectively diminish the occurrence of plaque, gingivitis and dental caries in youths at their late teens. The importance of social factors is also reported by *Färesjö et al.,* [20] while *others*[10, 34] presented the discussion around knowledge and attitudes related to dental health behaviour.

5. *Craft et al.* in the UK.[14, 15, 16] This study was directed towards the design and evaluation of community dental health education programmes. A controlled evaluation of a 3-week teacher-mediated dental health education curriculum package was undertaken in 35 secondary schools. About 4500 adolescents of 13–14 years were involved. Positive cognitive and affective changes were reported. Short-term behavioural changes were measured on plaque retention and longterm behavioural changes were measured on gingivitis scores. It was demonstrated that adolescents can be succesfully motivated to positively change their behaviour. This study may well be considered the largest trial of a dental health integrated

curriculum package ever conducted in Europe and is also unique from a methodological point of view.

6. *Schwartz et al.* in Denmark.[69, 76] In 1976, a preventive programme was established for young adults under the general dental programme of the Danish National Health Insurance. Almost 4000 persons received preventive services. Utilization, effects and feasibility were studied and information was collected on improvement of health status based on Visible Plaque Index and Gingival Bleeding Index. The service contained chairside dental education and discussion of and instruction in oral hygiene. Under the study conditions, a reduction of plaque and gingivitis by approximately 30% among those participating in the programme were recorded.

The programme should have clearly defined, time-related, measurable goals

The most common pitfalls in setting a health care goal are vagueness and over-optimism, or excessive ambition, the former leading to confusion, the latter to abandonment of the plan.[88]

An important step in planning preventive periodontal programmes at the community level is to define the priorities[9, 30] and to formulate a proper set of objectives. These objectives should be precise, responsive to the expressed demand rather than to the determined need, and stated in terms that are measurable and meaningful to dental and nondental personnel. They should also be understandable by political leaders and the public. For this latter purpose, the epidemiological and sociological terms should be translated into laymen's terms.[84]

The more precise and understandable the goals, the more helpful they will be. In the past, only a few rather vague goals were sometimes (mostly implicite) mentioned in official documents. Most of these were only expressed in terms of activities and then again in terms of activities of dental health workers, almost exclusively dentists.

Oral health goals can be precise and should be stated in terms of effects to be obtained, or expected results, and not in terms of activities. They should also be related to the coverage of the population. Furthermore, to disease measurement or better, *health* measurement because positive indicators (e. g. percentage of persons free of disease or percentage of persons with a functioning natural dentition) are preferred.

The major breakthrough in this problem area has been reached through WHO efforts. The World Health Assembly has, in 1979, adopted a resolution calling for the attainment of better health. The establishment of defined health goals has been encouraged by launching the slogan: *Health for All by the Year 2000.*[21, 89]

In 1981, the World Health Assembly adopted, as the first global indicator of oral health status, an average of not more than three decayed, missing, filled permanent teeth at the age of 12 by the year 2000. Further global goals related to dental caries and its sequelae are already proposed by WHO and FDI in terms of average number of teeth lost, or the percentage of edentulousness, or both.[21] Through collaborated efforts of WHO and the Commission on Oral Research and Epidemiology of the FDI, global goals for periodontal health in the year 2000 are now under consideration.[22] Defining health goals must be considered an innovative way to better oral health and it will be interesting to see their application to preventive periodontal programmes in the EEC.

The most important short-time goals seem to be in the area of health education – practising oral hygiene. Individual plaque control through self-care initiated by dental health education is, at the moment, the one and only solution we have. Longterm objectives are related to percentages of people free of disease or maintaining an adequate functioning dentition for life.

Goals should also recognize available resources and be realistic both in manpower and finances. Thus, it is advisable to reduce the goals to a level where the available resources are adequate instead of proposing over-ambitious goals.

The programme should be acceptable to the 'client' at the community level

The term 'client' at the community level is used here to indicate the (potential) consumers of a preventive periodontal programme in a broad sense, i.e. including health policy decision-makers, government agencies and those who regulate funding and resources. Thus, from individual persons to those in the political power circuit. A preventive periodontal programme should be connected to politically expressed demands and be relevant to the values, attitudes and behaviour of the population.

There has been only limited research on the specific, rather complex problem of implementation of preventive programmes in dentistry at the community level. An often heard critique is connected to the sometimes isolated attempts of dental care providers, who do not take into account or recognize the experience and expertise already available in other health care disciplines. The transfer of available technology into widespread use seems to be the most difficult part of the process. Some problem areas can be identified:

The scientific message is not accepted, nor the problem, or solution.

No matter how scientifically sound the message on the prevalence and the consequences of periodontal disease might be, dissonance occurs if the message is incompatible with a person's attitude, conviction or behaviour. The greater the difference between the views of the receiver and of the sender, the greater the dissonance experienced by the receiver. A large part of the population in Western Europe is not aware of the periodontal problem, let alone of the possibility of prevention. Also, these people do not know the advantages of such prevention.

Identifying the problem from a consumer's point of interest can be done following criteria for deciding the priority of problems according to a WHO document.[84] It can thus be stated that periodontal disease does threaten many people, and it can be prevented and controlled. But the condition is seldom of a emerging nature, as it is not causing great public concern because it is not causing death. Sequelae as tooth loss and edentulousness are not perceived by the public as threatening as many dental professionals tend to believe: a matter of wishful thinking?

Communities perceptions of periodontal health and prevention might not fit into the scientific solutions and available technology. Scientists, as well as the providers of care do have difficulty in identifying themselves with those they are ultimately working for. This is crucial for preventive periodontal programmes, where the only available technology today is individual self-care and oral hygiene through health education.

We still have a long way to go in health education and in promoting better oral hygiene. Only recently the old phrase 'Thou shalt' has been changed to 'Would you?', while it might be more appropriate to say 'Would we try together?'.[67]

One of the dangers of today is that, for instance, the results of the *Axelsson-Lindhe* studies in Karlstad in Sweden,[6] are too easily transposed to other settings in other countries, where such a programme might not be acceptable at all for several reasons.

Such an extensive programme might not be acceptable to society on the basis of cost analysis. One can elaborate in terms of effectiveness and efficiency, plus the attributes of interest, adequacy, availability, accessability, appropriateness and acceptability.[8, 60, 63, 71, 84] How much periodontal disease can be prevented at a cost which is acceptable to society?

To continue with client-centred barriers, plaque control through individual excersises might simply be too difficult or too much work for the rather vague, longterm rewards. But, in fact, we do not know what motivates people to exercise good oral hygiene and this question should be placed in the context in which oral health care is being delivered at present. However, there are promising trends: sales of toothbrushes have gone up tremendously in the last decade. The fast growing number of cases with toothbrush traumas presented at university clinics might be distressing, but nevertheless a sign of more attention for oral hygiene by the public.

Another current issue of debate is: by exactly what mechanism are plaque levels brought down in experimental clinical trials and in large groups of the population? Observations by, for instance, *Glavind et al.*[27, 28, 29] and *Söderholm et al.*[78, 79] in researching the necessary frequency and extend of professional prophylaxis and oral hygiene instruction have brought confusion on the research scene, but also more optimism on the feasibily of obtaining better oral hygiene at relatively low cost using less trained personnel.

A promising sign is also the fact that figures for caries prevalence and incidence in Western Europe are coming down. This phenomenon can at least partly be attributed to the widespread use of fluoride-containing toothpastes which in essence is self-care. A personal forecast is that within a decade toothpaste manufacturers will be able to include a substance in toothpaste which attacks the early plaque formation at the tooth-saliva interface. Such a technological innovation might help tremendously in preventive programmes at the community level.

In conclusion, the major thrust of periodontal prevention should be to increase public awareness about signs and symptoms of periodontal health and disease, and about the value and rewards of a personal preventive regime. Such a message should be placed in broad context, as oral health seems highly dependent on life style in general.

The programme should be relevant and acceptable at the professional level

In Europe the system for delivering dental health care is not client-centred, but build around the professional workers, in fact around the dentist. The dentist is the key person in the provision of care, and professional organizations of dentists comprise a main lobbying body within decision-making agencies and governmental circles, at both regional and national levels. As an example, look at the list of participants at this EEC Conference!

This phenomenon should be recognized before pursuing any major effort in dental health care. The relevance and acceptability for dentists (and also dental hygienists) are items to be discussed. A preventive periodontal programme that is threatening to the profession will never work; and 'threatening' means something that is *perceived* as a danger. It may be in the area of 'busyness', working conditions, or the possible type of work in the future, and there are implications for the profession when preventive periodontal programmes are introduced on a large scale. If we agree that the only feasible approach is dental health education and motivating self-care through oral hygiene, then the logical way is to use far less comprehensive trained personnel to perform a large part of the necessary professional work. Of course, a successful preventive programme will also generate a considerable demand for more sophisticated procedures and treatment. It will also imply that more teeth are retained longer into older age, being nevertheless 'at risk' to caries, fractures and periodontal disease. So when rational reasoning prevails, dentists need not be concerned about less business in the near future because of preventive programmes. How the dental profession perceives the above statements might be quite another story!

Many investigations have shown that traditional dental care, chiefly directed toward restorative treatment, does not prevent the gradual destruction of the dentition. It is also true that the prophylactic and periodontal areas of dental care systems are underutilized by the profession. It has, for instance, been demonstrated in the Netherlands that possibilities in the dental insurance system are only used by a few dentists, while it has also become fashionable for dentists to complain that periodontology and prevention is not covered by the national dental assurance system. It seems that the profession in itself is one of the barriers on the road towards better periodontal health. Some reasons for ignoring preventive/periodontal services have been indicated as follows:

- economic advantages in carrying out other services in the fee for item system;
- lack of knowledge on how preventive care could be carried out;
- historical organization of practice and the care system;
- the dentist is technically oriented and achieves job satisfaction by technical procedures;
- prevention does not give status, heroic treatment does indeed;
- the dentist is afraid of the soft, behavioural sciences area;
- prevention does not give visible results on short-term.

The education of the dentist is of critical importance.[23, 64] One cannot deny that the above attitudes of the profession must have grown during the educational years. The staff at the dental school with their own set of values, attitudes and behaviour do have a perhaps not easy to measure, but nevertheless tremendous influence on the future profession. According to Ainamo,[1] nothing short of a miracle should happen in dental schools to alter the educational environment for the future profession. But, on the other hand, why not a miracle? This is not impossible however as long as there is no conflict of interests between educators, providers and consumers of health care.[64]

Because it is possible and reasonable to employ less trained and less costly personnel in preventive periodontal programmes, there are now authorities in the field who would like to see a system where the dentist is not engaged in prevention at all. Other, less trained personnel should take over that part of the job completely. While such a move seems logical from a cost-effectiveness approach, the drawbacks are enormous. Because in such a system the dentists will be reinforced in their technical/curative approach and consequently the 'curative lobby' will prevent any further progress in prevention and in periodontal health.

The programme should include an evaluation and feedback system

Even the best planning is incomplete when a working procedure for control and evaluation is not included. The introduction and running of a preventive periodontal programme, without the possibility to closely follow the results, is not acceptable. Most experimental clinical trials today do have appropriate control groups and are closely supervised. But a large part of the care delivery in dentistry is without objective evaluation on results, cost analysis and proper feedback to the original objectives, if these are available at all.[8, 35, 60, 71, 88]

During the course of a large scale preventive periodontal programme, unexpected events might occur and alter the ultimate results. Also new knowledge and technology might emerge in the meantime which has to be implemented in the already existing programmes. So evaluation is mandatory in order to obtain a proper cycle of reevaluation, replanning and reprogramming. Also the use of a nationwide system of observing the patterns of oral health and disease must be advocated. Such a system could recognize changes in health and disease at the community level, which occur without any change in policies and without applying large scale programmes. To illustrate this point, the caries reduction wave has come to some European countries rather by surprise. It is thus difficult to trace the causative factors and use them in a positive way. One of the ways to use observed changes is the feedback into the planning of manpower. In several European countries the situation has arisen in which education and training of the different types of dental health workers and the prevalence of dental diseases do have opposite trends. That phenomenon could in itself become a barrier to the implementation of preventive periodontal programmes at the community level.

Conclusion. A Proposed Strategy

In conclusion, there is a recognized but not commonly accepted major public health problem. The scientific state of the art permits a firm basis for the solution. It is however difficult to formulate appropriate objectives related to the overall aim, while still recognizing available resources. Defining such goals will be a clear step forward. It has been shown that periodontal disease can be controlled effectively and that further loss of attachment can be arrested through special programmes for adolescents and adults. Whether such programmes are called prevention or therapy is a matter of semantics, because all programmes aim at the prevention of tooth loss and the ultimate goal is the natural functioning dentition for life: 'Enough teeth to smile, enough molars for stable comfort'. The choice should not only be acceptable to the client at the community level, but also relevant and acceptable to the dental profession.

The strong positive correlation between plaque and periodontal disease provides the only available target at present. If the population can be encouraged to improve their oral cleanliness, then the levels of periodontal disease will decrease. Therefore, the major thrust of activities should be in the area of mass plaque control:
- increase public awareness;
- develop planned health education;
- use social and educational strategies;
- encourage oral cleanliness.

Traditionally, health education has been the responsibility of public health agencies at the community level and of the individual dentist at the patient level. I would like to see a concerted effort of professional associations and governmental agencies to launch large scale preventive periodontal programmes in order to lower the amounts of plaque at the community level.

When such an effort is planned carefully and specifically to overcome the barriers at implementation, we all can look forward to better periodontal health by the year 2000.

References:

1. *Ainamo J.*
   The significance of periodontal disease in society. In Efficacy of Treatment Procedures in Periodontics. (Shanley D. ed.) Quintessence, Chicago, 1981: 299–316.

2. *Ainamo J., Barmes D., Beagrie G., Cutress T.* and *Martin J.*
Development of the World Health Organization (WHO) Community Periodontal Index of Treatment Needs (CPITN). Int. Dent. J., 1982, 32: 281–291.

3. *American Dental Association.*
Interim Report of the American Dental Association's Special Committee on the Future of Dentistry: Issue papers on dental research, manpower, education, practice and public and professional concerns. American Dental Association. Chicago, September 1982.

4. *American Dental Association.*
The Future of Dentistry. Progress report for the American Dental Association Open Hearing. Annual Meeting of the American Association of Dental Schools. New Orleans, March 1982.

5. *Anerud A., Löe H., Boysen H.* and *Smith M.*
The natural history of periodontal disease in man. Changes in gingival health and oral hygiene before 40 years of age. J. Periodontal. Res., 1979, 14: 526–540.

6. *Axelsson P.* and *Lindhe J.*
Effect of controlled oral hygiene procedures on caries and periodontal disease in adults. Results after 6 years. J. Clin. Periodontol., 1981, 8: 239–248.

7. *Badersten A., Nilvéus R.* and *Egelberg J.*
Effect of nonsurgical periodontal therapy. I. Moderately advanced periodontitis. J. Clin. Periodontol., 1981, 8: 57–72.

8. *Bailit H. L.*
Optimizing the dental delivery system. Int. Dent. J., 1982, 32: 65–73.

9. *Barenthin I.*
A review and discussion of goals in community dentistry. Community Dent. Oral Epidemiol., 1975, 3: 45–51.

10. *Bergendal B., Erasmie T.* and *Hamp S-E.*
Dental prophylaxis for youth in their late teens. III. Attitudes to teeth and dental health and their relation to dental health behavior. J. Clin. Periodontol., 1982, 9: 46–56.

11. *Björn A. L.*
Dental Health in relation to age and dental care. Thesis University of Lund. Odont. Revy., 1974, 25: suppl. 29.

12. *Björn A. L.*
Economy aspects of preventive dentistry. In Dental Health Care in Scandinavia. (Frandsen A. ed.) Quintessence, Chicago, 1982, 217–224.

13. *Bustad P.*
Communication and the prevention of dental diseases. In Preventive Dentistry in Practice. (Frandsen A. ed.) Munksgaard, Copenhagen 1976, 114–141.

14. *Craft M. H.* and *Croucher R. E.*
Preventive dental health in adolescents. Results of a controlled field trial. R. Soc. Health J., 1979, 2: 48–56.

15. *Craft M., Croucher R.* and *Dickinson J.*
Preventive dental health in adolescents: short and long term pupil response to trials of an integrated curriculum package. Community Dent. Oral Epidemiol., 1981, 9: 199–206.

16. *Craft M. H., Croucher R. E.* and *Dickinson J. A.*
Whole healthy or diseased disabled teeth? Health Education Council Monograph Series 4. The Health Education Council, London, 1981.

17. *Davies A. R.* and *Ware J. E.*
Measuring patient satisfaction with dental care. Soc. Sci. Med., 1981, 15A: 751–760.

18. *Department of Health and Social Security.*
Towards Better Dental Health: Guidelines for the future. The Report of the Dental Strategy Review Group. Department of Health and Social Security. London, 1981, 63 pp.

19. *Dwore R. B.* and *Krenter M. W.*
Update: Reinforcing the case for health promotion. J. Family Community Health., 1980, 2: 103–119.

20. *Färesjö, T. et al.*
Influence of social factors on the effect of different prophylactic regimens. Swed., Dent. J., 1981, 5; suppl. 7.

21. *Federation Dentaire International.*
Goals for Oral Health in the Year 2000. FDI Newsletter 1982, March, No. 122.

22. *Federation Dentaire International.*
Goals for Periodontal Health in the Year 2000. FDI-CORE Working Paper 1982, April.

23. *Frandsen A.*
Educational objectives in relation to provision of care. In Efficacy of Treatment Procedures in Periodontics. (Shanley D. ed.) Quintessence, Chicago, 1981, 257–272.

24. *Frazier P. J.*
A new look at dental health education in community programs. Dent. Hygiene, 1978, 52: 176–186.

25. *Frazier P. J.*
Social Factors of Dental Caries and Periodontal Disease: An Epidemiological Approach to Community Oral Health Education. Working Paper for

the WHO/FDI Scientific Workshop on Etiology and Prevention of Dental Caries and Periodontal Disease. WHO, Geneva, 1980.

26. *Frazier P. J.* and *Horowitz A. M.*
Priorities in planning and evaluating community oral health programs. J. Family Community Health, 1980, 3: 103–113.

27. *Glavind L.*
Effect of monthly professional mechanical tooth cleaning on periodontal health in adults. J. Clin. Periodontol., 1977, 4: 100–106.

28. *Glavind, L.* and *Attström, R.*
Periodontal self-examination. A motivational tool in periodontics. J. Clin. Periodontol., 1979, 6: 238–251.

29. *Glavind L., Zeuner E.* and *Attström R.*
Oral hygiene instruction of adults by means of a self-instructional manual. J. Clin. Periodontol., 1981, 8: 165–176.

30. *Gjermo P.*
Establishment of priorities in periodontal care. In Efficacy of treatment procedures in periodontics. (Shanley D. ed.) Quintessence, Chicago, 1981, 317–324.

31. *Håkanson J.* and *Söderholm G.*
Evaluation of dental health programmes for adults. In Dental Health Care in Scandinavia. (Frandsen A. ed.) Quintessence, Chicago, 1982, 107–120.

32. *Hamp S. E., Lindhe J., Fornell J., Johansson L. A.* and *Karlson R.*
Effect of a field program based on systematic plaque control on caries and gingivitis in school-children after 3 years. Community Dent. Oral Epidemiol., 1978, 6: 17–23.

33. *Hamp S. E.* and *Johansson L. A.*
Dental prophylaxis for youth in their late teens. I. Clinical effect of different preventive regimes on oral hygiene, gingivitis and dental caries. J. Clin. Periodontol., 1982, 9: 22–34.

34. *Hamp S. E., Bergendal B., Erasmie T., Lindström G.* and *Mellbring S.*
Dental prophylaxis for youth in their late teens. II. Knowledge about dental health and diseases and the relation to dental health behaviour. J. Clin. Periodontol., 1982, 9: 35–45.

35. *Helöe L. A., Haugejorden O.* and *Helöe B.*
The short and long term effects of organized public dental programs. J. Dent. Res., 1980, 59, Spec. issue D, part II: 2253–2258.

36. *Hetland L.* and *Midtun N.*
Effect of Oral Hygiene Instructions Given by

Paraprofessional Personnel. Thesis University of Bergen, 1978.

37. *Hetland L.*
A model for a 'Company Dental Health Service' built on prophylactic principles. In Dental Health Care in Scandinavia. (Frandsen A. ed.) Quintessence, Chicago, 1982, 237–243.

38. *Hetland L., Midtun N.* and *Kristoffersen T.*
Effect of oral hygiene instructions given by para-professional personnel. Community Dent. Oral Epidemiol., 1982, 10: 8–14.

39. *Horowitz A. M.* and *Frazier J. T.*
Effective public education for achieving oral health. J. Family Community Health, 1980, 3: 91–101.

40. *Hugoson A.* and *Koch G.*
Oral health in 1000 individuals aged 3–70 years in the community of Jönköping, Sweden. Swed. Dent. J., 1979, 3: 69–87.

41. *Hugoson A.* et al.
Dental health 1973 and 1978 in individuals aged 3–20 years in the community of Jönköping, Sweden. Swed. Dent., 1980, 4: 217–229.

42. *Hugoson A.*
Continuing training of dental care personnel. Swed. Dent J., 1981, 5: 65–76.

43. *Hugoson A., Koch G.* and *Rylander H.*
Prevalence and distribution of gingivitis-periodontitis in children and adolescents. Swed. Dent. J., 1981, 5: 91–103.

44. *Hugoson A.* and *Koch G.*
Development of a preventive dental care programme for children and adolescents in the county of Jönköping 1973–1979. Swed. Dent. J., 1981, 5: 159–172.

45. *Hugoson A.* and *Rylander H.*
Longitudinal study of periodontal status in individuals aged 15 years in 1973 and 20 years in 1978 in Jönköping, Sweden. Community Dent. Oral Epidemiol., 1982, 10: 37–42.

46. *Hugoson A.* and *Koch J.*
Dental Health 1973 and 1978 in individuals aged 3–20 years in the community of Jönköping, Sweden. In Dental Health Care in Scandinavia. (Frandsen A. ed.) Quintessence, Chicago, 1982, 225–231.

47. *Hugoson A.* and *Jordan T.*
Frequency distribution of individuals aged 20–70 years according to severity of periodontal disease. Community Dent. Oral Epidemiol., 1982, 10: 187–192.

48. *Käyser A. F.*
Shortened dental arches and oral function. J. Oral Rehabil., 1981, 8: 457–462.

49. *Kristofferson T.*
Evaluation of dental health programmes for adults. In Dental Health Care in Scandinavia. (Frandsen A. ed.) Quintessence, Chicago, 1982, 121–127.

50. *Lennon M. A., Downer M. C., O'Mullane D. M.* and *Taylor G. O.*
The role of community clinical trials in public health decisions in preventive dentistry. J. Dent. Res., 1980, 59, Spec. issue: D, part II 2243–2247.

51. *Lindhe J., Westfelt E., Nyman S., Socransky S. S., Heijl L.* and *Bratthall G.*
Healing following surgical/non-surgical treatment of periodontal disease. A clinical study. J. Clin. Periodontol., 1982, 9: 115–128.

52. *Lindhe J., Socransky S. S., Nyman S., Haffajee A.* and *Westfelt E.*
'Critical probing depths' in periodontal therapy. J. Clin. Periodontal., 1982, 9: 323–336.

53. *Listgarden M. H.* and *Levine S.*
Positive correlations between the proportions of subgingival spirochetes and motile bacteria and susceptibility of human subjects to periodontal deterioration. J. Clin. Periodontol., 1981, 8: 122–138.

54. *Listgarten M.* and *Schifter C.*
Differential dark field microscopy of subgingival bacteria as an aid in selecting recall intervals: results after 18 months. J. Clin. Periodontol., 1982, 9: 305–316.

55. *Morrison E. C., Ramfjord S. P.* and *Hill R. W.*
Short-term effects of initial nonsurgical periodontal treatment (hygienic phase). J. Clin. Periodontol., 1980, 7: 199–211.

56. *O'Mullane D. M.*
Efficiency in clinical trials of caries preventive agents and methods. Community Dent. Oral Epidemiol., 1976, 4: 190–194.

57. *Nuffield Foundation.*
An Inquiry into Dental Education. A report to the Nuffield Foundation. London 1980, 115 pp.

58. *Parsby, J. E.*
Communication and behavioural change. In Preventive Dentistry in Practice. (Frandsen A. ed.) Munksgaard, Copenhagen 1976, 92–113.

59. *Philstrom B. L., Ortiz-Campos C.* and *McHugh R. B.*
A randomized four-year study of periodontal therapy. J. Periodontol., 1981, 52: 5: 227–242.

60. *Pilot T.* and *Sheiham A.*
Beoordeling van het resultaat van tandheelkundige verzorging in Nederland. Ned. Tijdschr. Tandheelkd., 1977, 84: 224–234.

61. *Pilot T.*
Pleidooi tegen het verlengen van de verkorte tandboog. Ned. Tijdschr. Tandheelkd., 1978, 85: 477–480.

62. *Pilot T.* and *Schaub R. M. H.*
Barriers preventing the application of present knowledge of prevention and therapy to the Dutch population. J. Clin. Periodontol., 1980, 7: 347.

63. *Pilot T.*
Analysis of the overall effectiveness of treatment of periodontal disease. In Efficacy of Treatment Procedures in Periodontics. (Shanley D. ed.) Quintessence, Chicago, 1981, 213–230.

64. *Pilot T.*
Staff development to meet future needs of dental education. Tidskr. Odontol. Pedagogik., 1982, 5: 21–25.

65. *Rayant G. A.* and *Sheiham A.*
An analysis of factors affecting compliance with tooth-cleaning recommendations. J. Clin. Periodontol., 1980, 7: 289–299.

66. *Reisine S. T.*
Theoretical considerations in formulating sociodental indicators. Soc. Sci. Med., 1981, 15A: 745–750.

67. *Rouwenhorst W.* Gezondheidsvoorlichting en -opvoeding, toen en nu. Paper presented at the symposium ter gelegenheid van het emeriaat van Prof. Dr. O. Backer Dirks, October, 1982.

68. *Schaub R. M. H.*
Barriers to Effective Periodontal Care. Paper presented to the CORE working group 6, Periodontal diseases at the Annual World Dental Congress, FDI. Vienna, October, 1982.

69. *Schwarz E.*
Longitudinal evaluation of a preventive program provided by general dental practitioners to young adult Danes. Community Dent. Oral Epidemiol., 1981, 9: 280–284.

70. *Selikowitz H-S., Sheiham A., Albert D.* and *Williams G. M.*
Retrospective longitudinal study of the rate of alveolar bone loss in humans using bite-wings radiographs. J. Clin. Periodontol., 1981, 8: 431–438.

71. *Sheiham A.*
An evaluation of the success of dental care in the

United Kingdom. Brit. Dent. J.; 1973, 135: 271–279.

72. *Sheiham A.*
Screening for periodontal disease. J. Clin. Periodontol., 1978, 5: 237–245.

73. *Sheiham A.*
Current concepts in health education. In Efficacy of Treatment Procedures in Periodontics. (Shanley D. ed.) Quintessence, Chicago 1981, 23–40.

74. *Sheiham A.*
Promoting periodontal health – effective programmes of education and promotion. Int. Dent. J., 1983, 33: 182–187

75. *Singletary M. M., Crawford J. J.* and *Simpson D. M.*
Dark field microscopic monitoring of subgingival bacteria during periodontal therapy. J. Periodontol., 1982, 53: 671–687.

76. *Skougaard M.*
Evaluation of dental health programmes for adults. In Dental Health Care in Scandinavia. (Frandsen A. ed.) Quintessence, Chicago, 1982, 129–132.

77. *Söderholm G.*
Effect of a Dental Care Programme on Dental Health Conditions. A study of employees of a Swedish Shipyard. Thesis University of Lund, 1979.

78. *Söderholm G., Nobréus N., Attström R.* and *Egelberg J.*
Teaching plaque control. I. A five-visit versus a two-visit program. J. Clin. Periodontol., 1982, 9: 203–213.

79. *Söderholm G.* and *Egelberg J.*
Teaching plaque control. II. 30-minute versus 15-minute appointments in a three-visit program. J. Clin. Periodontol., 1982, 9: 214–222.

80. *Waerhaug J.*
What is the objective of treatment: disease elimination, control or reduction? In Efficacy of Treatment Procedures in Periodontics. (Shanley D. ed.) Quintessence, Chicago, 1981, 235–244.

81. *WHO.*
Statistical Indicators for the planning and evaluation of public health programmes. Fourteenth Report of the WHO Expert Commitee on Health Statistics. WHO Technical Report Series No. 472. WHO Geneva, 1971, 40 pp.

82. *WHO.*
Planning and evaluation dental health services. Report of a Working Group, EURO 5505. WHO Regional Office for Europe, Copenhagen, 1972, 41 pp.

83. WHO.
The application of epidemiology to the planning and evaluation of health services. Report of a Working Group, EURO 4905. WHO Regional Office for Europe, Copenhagen, 1974, 25 pp.

84. *WHO.*
Planning and evaluation of public dental health services. Report of a WHO Expert Commitee. WHO Technical Report Series No. 589. WHO, Geneva, 1976, 33 pp.

85. *WHO.*
Epidemiology, etiology and prevention of periodontal diseases. Report of a WHO Expert Committee. WHO Technical Report Series No. 621. WHO, Geneva, 1978, 60 pp.

86. *WHO.*
Primary health care. Report of the International Conference of Primary Health Care. WHO, Geneva 1978.

87. *WHO.*
Principles and methods of health education. European Report Series No. 11. WHO, Copenhagen, 1979.

88. *WHO.*
Planning oral health services. Offset Publication No. 53. WHO, Geneva, 1980, 49 pp.

89. *WHO.*
Plan of action for implementing the global strategy for Health for All. Health for All series No. 7. WHO, Geneva, 1982.

15. Longitudinal Data on Practice-Based Preventive Periodontal Care

Göran Söderholm and Rolf Attström

Introduction

In the last two decades many studies have been published in relation to the prevalence of periodontal disease. Although knowledge of the aetiology and pathogenesis of periodontal disease has expanded, there is little increase in the amount of convincing epidemiological data. Some of the studies are confusing and contradictory because of unclear definitions and minimal differences between the criteria. Nevertheless, it is possible to state that the frequency and severity of periodontitis increase with advancing age.[1, 2, 7, 14, 29, 31] In Figure 15.1, from the study by *Björn,*[7] the relationship between bone loss and patient's age is illustrated. A higher score indicates more loss of periodontal attachment. In the study by *Sheiham* in 1969,[31] it was shown that 48% of an adult population were in the terminal stage of periodontal disease. For individuals between 45 and 49 years, 79% were in the terminal stage of periodontal disease. The proportion of individuals with periodontal pockets greater than 4 mm increases from 10% in the age group 20–24 years to 50% in the highest age group.

The rate of bacteria in periodontal disease is well-documented in several studies (see reviews by *Socransky*[34] and *Slots*[32]). Thus, a positive correlation between accumulation of plaque and presence of periodontal disease has been repeatedly demonstrated, e.g. *Schei.*[29]

Longitudinal Studies

Expanding knowledge of the prevalence of periodontal disease, its role in the loss of teeth, and the role of microbes in the aetiology of the disease has initiated longitudinal studies aimed at preventing the disease.[3, 4, 10, 11, 12, 13, 15, 16, 19, 21, 25, 28, 35, 36] The common factor in the different dental health care programmes in all these studies is recall of the patients for repeated 'plaque control'. The content of the 'plaque control' visits varies from study to study, but always includes scaling, curettage, polishing and root planing. Intentionally or not, these programmes also gradually change the patient's attitude and behaviour in a positive way with respect to their dental health.[10] Patients participating in such programmes improve their oral hygiene procedures, change their diet habits and often choose fluoride dentifrices; The interval between recall visits varies from a visit every two weeks to one every 6 months. The effects of the different programmes are described for the following parameters:

1. The effect on oral hygiene.
2. The effect on attachment loss.
3. The effect on tooth mortality rate.

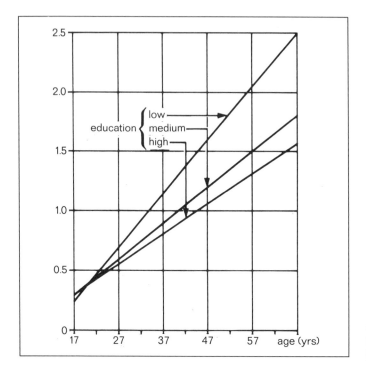

Fig. 15.1 Regression of bone scores on age, staff members (Björn[7]).

Oral hygiene

In the study by *Löe et al*,[21] a Norwegian population of 565 male students between 17 and 30 years were compared with another group from Sri Lanka consisting of 480 male tea labourers between 15 and 30 years of age. Over 90% of the Norwegian group up to the age of 14 years participated in a programme, incorporating supervised brushing with the application of 0.2% sodium fluoride 4 times per year. From grade 1 through 7, they also received individual instruction or re-instruction in oral hygiene techniques once a year. Of the children from 3 to 23 years of age, 90% had participated in programmes consisting of examinations and treatment on an annual recall schedule. After the age of 23, a very welldeveloped system of private practitioners, with the ratio of 1 dentist per 600 patients, was available.

The Sri Lankan group consisted of tea labourers who had never been exposed to any prevention or treatment for dental diseases.

For comparison of the oral hygiene status, Plaque Index (Pl I, Silness and Löe) was used. In the Norwegian group, 64% of the surfaces scored had a plaque index of one or less, compared with only 4% in the Sri Lankan group (Fig. 15.2).

Studies concerning the effect of different self-instruction programmes on oral hygiene and gingival health have been made by *Glavind* and *co-workers*.[11, 12, 13] In one of the studies[13] the purpose was to determine the applicability of self-instructional materials for oral hygiene instruction to general dental practice. The results indicated that a self-instructional programme was almost as effective as person-to-person instruction (Fig. 15.3). *Axelsson* and *Lindhe*[3] present data after 6 years con-

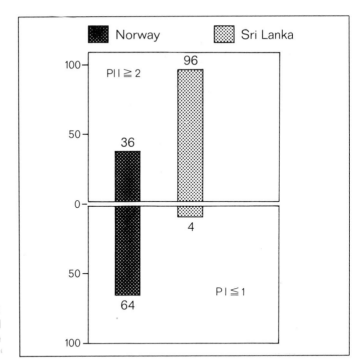

Fig. 15.2 PII ≥2 and PII ≤1 scores (%) Norwegians and Sri Lankans at baseline 1969–1970 (Löe *et al*[21]).

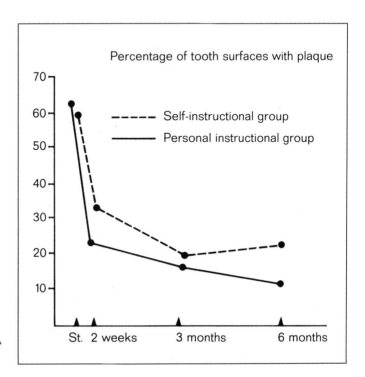

Fig. 15.3 Mean plaque scores of the treatment groups at the examinations during the period of treatment (Glavind *et al*[11–13]).

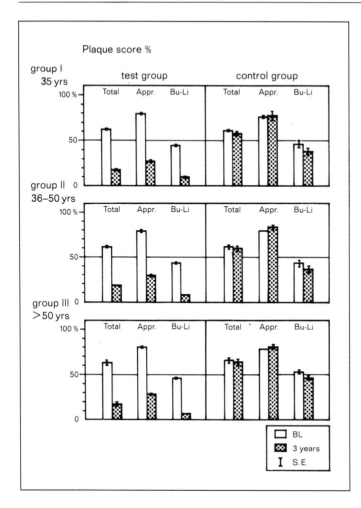

Fig. 15.4 Histogram describing the frequency distribution of tooth surfaces harboring plaque at the baseline examination and at 3 and 6 years later (Axelsson and Lindhe[3]).

trolled oral hygiene procedures. There were 310 individuals in the test group, and 146 in the control group. The test group received a preventive treatment repeated every 2–3 months. The control group were not involved in any dental health programme, but were called in for symptomatic dental treatment once a year.

The initial mean plaque surfaces were between 60–70% in both groups and were reduced to between 15–20% in test patients. The control patients did not im-

prove during the 6 years of treatment (Fig. 15,4).

In the study by Söderholm,[36] 256 white-collar workers and 198 blue-collar workers were examined during a period of 13 years. A dental health programme was performed during the last 4 years of this period. The maintenance care programme consisted of recalls for 'plaque control' every 3rd month. Initially, white as well as blue-collar workers had between 60–70% tooth surfaces covered with plaque. They

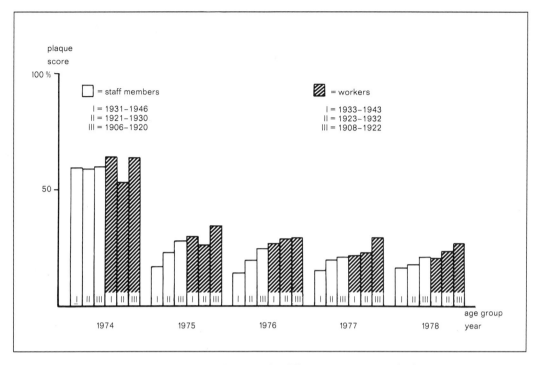

Fig. 15.5 Mean plaque scores for participants in different age groups before treatment (1974) and throughout the experimental period (Söderholm[36]).

reduced plaque and improved their oral hygiene during the test period. After 4 years, the number of surfaces with plaque were between 20% and 30% per individual (Fig. 15.5). The percentages of surfaces with plaque at the three examination times for individuals in the three age groups are illustrated in Figure 15.6.

A series of studies concerning periodontal surgery and maintenance care[4, 16, 18, 19] show that repeated professional tooth cleaning every 2 weeks during the first 2 months, and then every 3rd month, resulted in Plaque Index (plaque index *Sillness* and *Löe*) consistently close to O after test periods of 2–3 years.

In 1977, *Suomi* and *co-workers*[35] published a longitudinal study on 'The effect of controlled oral hygiene procedures on the progression of periodontal disease in adults'. During the first year, 216 test patients received professional oral prophylaxis at 2, 4, 6, and 9 month intervals, at 3 month intervals during the 2nd year, and at 4 months intervals during the 3rd year. The 263 matched individuals in the control groups received no preventive maintenance dental care. Mean debris scores for experimental groups decreased slightly from baseline. In control groups debris scores increased.

In summary, all studies attempting to treat and prevent periodontal diseases were based on recall plaque control programmes, aimed at the removal of microbial plaque from the tooth surfaces. The frequencies of recall varied from once every 14 days to once every 6 months.

201

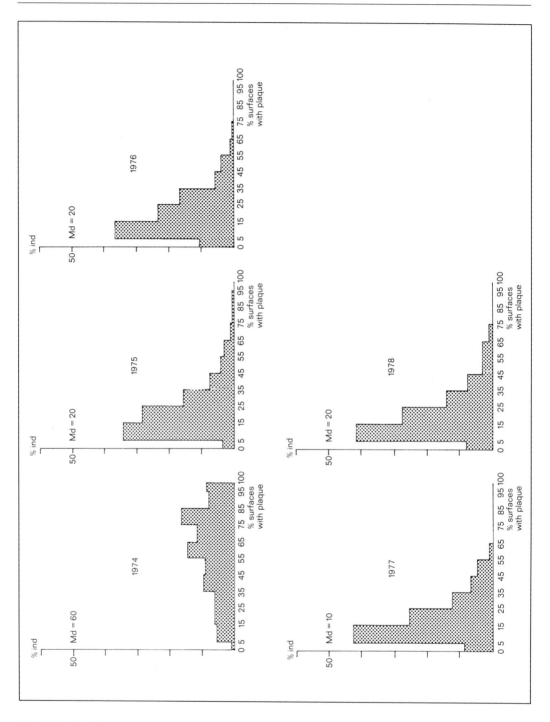

Fig. 15.6 Distribution of percentage staff members on different plaque scores before treatment (1974) and throughout the experimental period (Söderholm[36]).

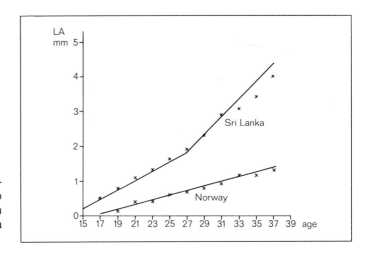

Fig. 15.7 Annual rate of attachment loss in those who participated in all surveys in Norway and Sri Lanka (Löe[23]).

The recall visits in some studies consisted of professional cleaning and in others only self-instructional manuals were provided. They all improved oral hygiene based on scores using different plaque indicies. The decrease in plaque scores were maintained.

Attachment loss

Longitudinal data can reveal the severity and rate of progression of periodontal disease. If we wish to evaluate the effects of preventive periodontal care, then longitudinal data will also be necessary. With regard to pocket depth and attachment loss these can be measured clinically using a periodontal probe. The methodological variables were recently described by *Fowler et al.*[9] To attain acceptable reproducability in these parameters, it is necessary to use a standardized probing pressure and a constant reference point in relation to changes in probing attachment levels.

Another way to measure attachment level is to estimate bone level as a percentage of the total length of the teeth on x-rays,

described by *Björn.*[8] In the study by *Löe et al,*[22] the loss of attachment was studied over 6 years. The material and oral hygiene programmes are described above. A blunt probe with a diameter of 0.6 mm and graded at 1, 2, 3, 4, 5, 7, 9 and 11 mm were used.

The results indicate that the mean annual rate of attachment loss for the Norwegian group approaching 40 years of age was 0.08 mm for interproximal surfaces. Comparable data for the Sri Lankan group was 0.30 mm (Fig. 15.7). The authors also state that the periodontal lesion progresses continuously.

In the longitudinal study by *Axelsson* and *Lindhe,*[3] attachment levels were observed over 6 years. Materials and preventive programmes are described above.

In the test groups no further loss of attachment during the 6 year period were recorded. The average attachment loss per year was in control groups I: 0.13 mm, II: 0.23 mm and in III: 0.26 mm.

Söderholm[36] presented longitudinal data from 413 patients for bone height measured from orthopantomograms. During the first 9 years, the patients received traditional dental care and for the last 4 years

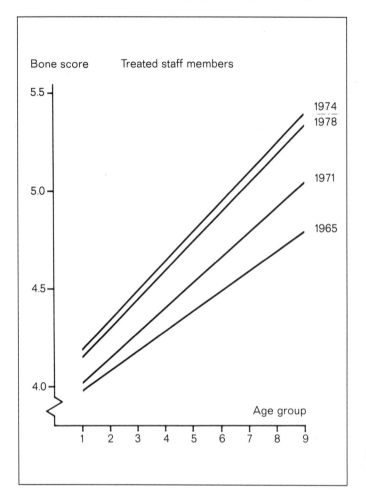

Fig. 15.8 Regression of bone scores on age (Söderholm[36]).

they were given the above described maintenance care.

During the traditional care period, the medians of bone scores increased from 4.25–4.71 in white collar workers and from 4.60–4.86 in blue-collar workers. During the maintenance care period a slight improvement in bone score level was noted (Fig. 15.8). If the bone level changes are expressed in millimeters, the annual attachment loss during the traditional care period would be about 0.03 mm per year in the youngest groups and 0.30 mm/year in the oldest groups.

Several studies have been made with the purpose of evaluating the effect of different surgical methods, combined with maintenance care in moderate and advanced periodontitis.[4, 15, 19, 28] They all demonstrated success in preventing further loss of attachment in patients with active periodontitis. At the same time it seemed to be minor differences between different surgical methods, provided that an adequate maintenance care was carried out. However, in the study by *Lindhe et al.*,[20] attachment loss occurred in situations with initial shallow pockets as an effect of surgical trauma.

Selikowitz et al.[30] presented data from a retrospective longitudinal study on the rate of alveolar bone loss in humans using bite-wing radiographs. Over 10 years, 100 pairs of bite-wings were analysed. The patients had been given a regular systematic scaling, polishing and health education every 3 to 6 months. The average vertical bone loss per year was between 0.3 mm – 0.05 mm, depending on which reference point was used.

Suomi[35] presented data on attachment level changes as a function of controlled oral hygiene. The experimental groups lost less than 0.03 mm attachment per year, compared with control groups without maintenance care where the attachment loss was about 0.10 mm per year per individual.

In summary, all studies attempting to treat and prevent periodontal disease were successful. After treatment the yearly attachment loss rate was less than 0.08 mm per year and was zero in most cases. Controls demonstrate up to 0.30 mm attachment loss per year.

Tooth mortality

The primary purpose of dental treatment is to provide the patients with such care that will retain enough teeth to satisfy functional and aesthetical requirements. We know that periodontal diseases are responsible for a great number of extractions. We need to demonstrate the effectiveness of the preventative programmes on tooth mortality. Because of the very slow progression of the disease (only about average of 0.2 mm attachment loss per year), it is necessary to have a very long test period in order to be sure of the effectiveness of the programme.

Hirschfeld and *Wassermann*[15] presented retrospective data about tooth loss in 600 patients. The patients had received differing levels of surgical and reparative care, but all had received maintenance care at 4 to 6 month intervals. The average period of maintenance was 22 years. Three hundred patients lost no teeth from periodontal disease. In all, 8.3% of the teeth were lost. Periodontal causes led to the extraction of 7.1% of the total. From the 2139 teeth originally designated to have a questionable prognosis, 666 teeth were lost. Tooth loss seemed to be bilaterally symmetrical, tooth retention seemed more closely related to the individual case than the treatment modality employed.

In the study by *Löe* and *co-workers*,[23] tooth mortality over 6 to 7 years was investigated. The average number of teeth per person in the Norwegian group was 27.22. During the 7 year observation, 27 teeth (17 molars and 10 bicuspids) were lost among 245 individuals who participated in both the first (1969) and the last (1975) examinations. The 27 teeth lost were from 16 individuals, of these one tooth was lost due to periodontal disease. The mean number of teeth lost per individuals per year was 0.02.

The average number of teeth per person in the Sri Lankan group was 27.05. During the 7 year observation, 169 teeth (121 molars, 16 bicuspids and 32 incisors) were lost among 228 individuals. The teeth lost were from 77 individuals. The mean number of teeth lost per individual per year was 0.1 (Table 15.1).

In the study by *Söderholm*,[36] tooth mortality was monitored over approximately 13 years. The average number of teeth at the first examination was 25.1 for 256 white-collar workers and 21.9 for 189 blue-collar workers. After 9 years of traditional dental care, the average number of teeth for the white-collar workers and blue-collar workers were reduced to 23.5 and 19.8, respectively. Thus, the mean rate of tooth loss became 0.17 and 0.23 tooth per year.

Table 15.1 The number and types of tooth loss in Norway during 1969–1975 and Sri Lanka during 1970–1977 (Löe[23]).

Populations	Number indivi- duals	Number teeth lost	Molars	Bicuspids	Incisors
Norwegian students and academicians	245	27	17	10	
Sri Lankan tea labourers	228	169	121	16	32

During the 4 years of maintenance, the rate of lost teeth per year was 0.1 for both white- and blue-collar workers.

In summary, the studies referred to above demonstrate a lower number of teeth lost per year in the test groups subjected to preventive dental care. These results are discussed below.

Discussion

Several longitudinal studies describe the development of gingivitis and periodontitis. It is, however, impossible to predict the onset of destructive periodontitis. In spite of differences in programmes provided, all studies using repeated preventive care improved oral hygiene. The frequency of recall for prophylactic procedures has been a choice for the individual clinician. However, recently a series of studies[18, 23, 26] have shown clear-cut differences in the subgingival microflora before and after subgingival scaling. In the study by Mosques,[26] coccoid forms increased from 25% to 75% of the subgingival flora 3 days after scaling. Spirochaetes decreased from 34% to a low of 2% and returned to the baseline proportion after 42 days. In the study by Slots,[33] the proportion of spirochaetes returned to baseline only after 6 months. These results strongly confirm the value of frequently repeated preventing care every 3 to 6 months.

In an attempt to predict periodontal deterioration, Listgarten and Levin,[17] studied the correlation between the proportions of subgingivalspirochaetes and motile bacteria versus susceptibility of human subjects to periodontal deterioration. A positive correlation was established between the percentage of motile rods versus gingival index (GI) and plaque index (PI I) (Silness and Löe 1964) and between spirochaetes versus PI I and pocket depth. The authors conclude that the proportion of spirochaetes and motile rods in a pooled sample of subgingival debris is a good predictor of the likelihood that one or more teeth will deteriorate clinically within the next one year period. However, if pooled sample of debris are used, there must be a risk that one or several pockets with large proportions of spirochaetes will be overlooked. A safe way to prevent periodontal disease is still to have all individuals receive the maintenance care.

Regarding attachment loss in the control groups, all available data reveals a slow progression of about 0.2 mm attachment loss per year. However, during a period of 10 years, 2 mm loss of attachment will put some teeth in a threatened situation by spread of the disease process to, for example, furcation involvement. It is also necessary to know that every tooth extracted because of advanced periodontal disease in longitudinal studies will make the data about attachment loss more favourable than it actually is for the remaining teeth. This makes it necessary in all longitudinal studies to present data on attachment levels with regard to tooth mortality.

The final and most valuable measurement of our effectiveness in the treatment of patients is, of course, tooth mortality. However, cross-sectional data of tooth mortality that show a decrease in the number of teeth with increasing age not only reflects diseases that the patients have been subjected to, but also the following:

1. Attitudes of patients towards dental health.
2. Attitudes of dentists.
3. Availability of dental care.
4. Economic structures.
5. Geographical considerations.

In longitudinal studies one will notice that teeth remain for a long period though the periodontal disease progresses. In the Sri Lankan group in the study by *Löe et al,*[23] e.g. the yearly loss of teeth was not more than 0.1 teeth compared with another study by *Becker et al*[5] of untreated periodontal disease, the tooth loss per patient and per year was 0.61.

Once a longitudinal study has started, it will be necessary to take into consideration teeth extracted because of periodontal disease if we want to be sure about the rate of attachment loss. Given these conditions, a low rate of attachment loss, demonstrated in, for example, the studies by *Suomi, Axelsson, Söderholm, Löe*[3, 21, 35, 36] will probably not cause tooth loss to any great extent. However, data from a larger number of teeth over a very long time (30 years or more) is the only way of evaluating desired effectiveness of dental care.

General Considerations

During the last 15 years, several longitudinal studies with the goal of treating and preventing periodontal diseases have been started and are still going on. They are based on frequently repeated 'plaque control' and are providing the participants with an improved oral hygiene. The attachment loss is insignificant. The tooth mortality rate is decreased, but further information from these studies is needed.

Future Objectives

Most of the countries in the western world are suffering from economic crises. This considered, it is of great importance to carry out cost-effectiveness studies of continously performed maintenance care. Dental health care programmes have to be compared with traditional care, not only with respect to dental health but also to costs.

References

1. *Ainamo J.* and *Alvesalo L.*
   Periodontal conditions in a Finnish rural population. Acta. Odontol. Scand., 1968, 26: 489–500.

2. *Axelsson P., Göland U., Hugoson A., Koch G., Paulander J., Pettersson S., Rasmusson C.-G., Schmidt G.* and *Thilander H.*
   Tandhälsotillståndet hos 1000 personer i åldrarna 3 till 70 år inom Jönköpings kommun. II. Klinisk undersökning av hälsotillståndet hos tänder och käkar samt förekomst av protetiska rekonstruktioner. Tandläkartidningen, 1975, 67: 11–22.

3. *Axelsson P.* and *Lindhe J.*
   Effect of controlled oral hygiene procedures on caries and periodontal disease in adults. J. Clin. Periodontol., 1981, 8: 239–248.

4. *Badersten A., Nilvéus R.* and *Egelberg J.*
   Effect of non-surgical periodontal therapy. I. Moderately advanced periodontitis. J. Clin. Periodontol., 1981, 8:57–72.

5. *Becker W., Berg L.* and *Becker B. E.*
Untreated periodontal disease: a longitudinal study. J. Periodontol., 1979, 50: 234–244.

6. *Bergman B., Hugoson A.* and *Olsson C-O.*
Caries and periodontal status in patients fitted with removable partial dentures. J. Clin. Periodontol., 1977, 4: 134–146.

7. *Björn H.*
Tandhälsotillståndet hos manliga anställda vid en svensk industri. Tandläkartidningen, 1971, 63: 4–21.

8. *Björn A-L., Björn H.* and *Halling A.*
An abbreviated index for periodontal bone height. Odontol. Revy., 1975, 26: 225.

9. *Fowler C., Garrett S., Crigger M.* and *Egelberg J.*
Histologic probe position in treated and untreated human periodontal tissues. J. Clin. Periodontol., 1982, 9: 373–385.

10. *Glavind L.*
Effect of monthly professional mechanical tooth cleaning on periodontal health in adults. J. Clin. Periodontol., 1977, 4: 100–106.

11. *Glavind L.* and *Attström R.*
Periodontal self-examination. A motivation tool in periodontics. J. Clin. Periodontol., 1979, 6: 238–251.

12. *Glavind L., Zeuner E.* and *Attström R.*
Oral hygiene instructions of adults by means of a self-instructional manual. J. Clin. Periodontol., 1981, 8: 165–176.

13. *Glavind L., Pedersen E., Christensen H.* and *Attström R.*
Self-instructional material used in general dental practice for oral home care instruction. J. Clin. Periodontol. (In press).

14. *Håkansson J.*
Dental care habits, attitudes towards dental health and dental status among 20–60-year-old individuals in Sweden. Thesis. 1978. University of Lund, Sweden.

15. *Hirschfeld L.* and *Wasserman B.*
A long term survey of tooth loss in 600 treated periodontal patients. J. Periodontol., 1978, 49: 225–237.

16. *Knowles J. W., Burgett F. G., Nissle R. R., Shick R. A., Morrison E. C.* and *Ramfjord A. A.*
Results of periodontal treatment related to pocket depth and attachment level. Eight years. J. Periodontol., 1979, 50: 225–233.

17. *Listgarten M. J.* and *Levine S.*
Positive correlation between the proportions of subgingival spirochetes and motile bacteria and susceptibility of human subjects to periodontal deterioration. J. Clin. Periodontol., 1981, 8: 122–138.

18. *Listgarten M. A., Lindhe J.* and *Helldén L.*
Effect of tetracycline and/or scaling on human periodontal disease. Clinical microbiological and histological observations. J. Clin. Periodontol., 1981, 5: 246–271.

19. *Lindhe J.* and *Nyman S.*
The effect of plaque-control and surgical pocket elimination on establishment and maintenance of periodontal health. J. Clin. Periodontol., 1975, 2: 67–79.

20. *Lindhe J., Socransky S. S., Nyman S., Haffajee A.* and *Westfelt E.*
'Critical probing depths' in periodontal therapy. J. Clin. Periodontol., 1982, 9: 323–336.

21. *Löe H., Ånerud Å., Boysen H.* and *Smith M. R.*
The natural history of periodontal disease in man. Study design and base line data. J. Periodontal Res., 1978, 13: 550–562.

22. *Löe H., Ånerud Å., Boysen H.* and *Smith M. R.*
The natural history of periodontal disease in man. The rate of periodontal attachment before 40 years of age. J. Periodontol., 1978, 49: 607–620.

23. *Löe H., Ånerud Å., Boysen H.* and *Smith M. R.*
The natural history of periodontal disease in man. Tooth mortality rates before 40 years of age. J. Periodontal Res., 1978, 13: 563–572.

24. *Lövdal A., Arno A.* and *Waerhaug J.*
Incidence of clinical manifestations of periodontal disease in light of oral hygiene and calculus formation. J. Amer. Dent. Assoc., 1958, 56: 21–33.

25. *Lövdal A., Arno A., Schei O.* and *Waerhaug J.*
Combined effect of subgingival scaling and controlled oral hygiene on the incidence of gingivitis. Acta Odontol. Scand., 1961, 19: 537–555.

26. *Mousques T., Listgarten M. A.* and *Philips R. W.*
Effect of scaling and root planing on the composition of the human subgingival microbial flora. J. Periodont. Res., 1980, 15: 144–151.

27. *Petersen P. E.*
Tandplejeadfaerd, tandstatus og odontologisk behandlingsbehov blandt arbejdere og funktionaerer på en stor dansk industrivirksamhed. En social odontologisk bedriftsundersøgelse. Thesis. 1981.

28. *Rosling B., Nyman S.* and *Lindhe J.*
The effect of systematic plaque control on bone regeneration in infrabony pockets. J. Clin. Periodontol, 1976, 3: 38–53.

29. *Schei O., Waerhaug J., Lövdal A.* and *Arno A.*
Alveolar bone loss as related to oral hygiene and age. J. Periodontol., 1959: 30: 7–16.

30. *Selikowitz H.-S., Sheiham A., Albert D.* and *Williams G. M.*
Retrospective longitudinal study of the rate of alveolar bone loss in humans using bite-wing radiographs. J. Clin. Periodontol, 1981, 8: 431–439.

31. *Sheiham A.*
The prevalence and severity of periodontal disease in British populations. Dental surveys of employed populations in Great Britain. Brit. Dent. J., 1969, 126: 115–122.

32. *Slots J.*
Subgingival microflora and periodontal disease. J. Clin. Periodontol., 1979, 6: 351–382.

33. *Slots J., Mashimo P., Levine M. J.* and *Genco R. J.*
Periodontal therapy in humans. I. Microbiological and clinical effects of a single course of periodontal scaling and root planing and of adjunctive tetracycline therapy. J. Periodontol., 1979, 50: 495–509.

34. *Socransky S. S.*
Microbiology of periodontal disease. Present status and future considerations. J. Periodontol. 1977, 48: 497–504.

35. *Suomi J. D., Greene J. C. Vermillion J. R., Doyle J., Chang J. J.* and *Leatherwood E. C.*
The effect of controlled oral hygiene procedures on the progression of periodontal disease in adults: results after third and final year. J. Periodontol., 1971, 42: 152–160.

36. *Söderholm G.*
Effect of a dental care program on dental health conditions. A study of employees of a Swedish Shipyard. Thesis. 1979. University of Lund, Sweden.

16. The Identification of Teenage Children at High Risk to Periodontal Disease

Michael A. Lennon and Valerie Clerehugh

Introduction

At the last workshop on *The efficacy of treatment procedures in periodontics* in 1979, *Gjermo*[3] suggested that the control of periodontal disease could be considered at three levels. Firstly, primary prevention to maintain periodontal health, secondly the detection and treatment of early disease and, thirdly, the treatment of established disease. This review is concerned with the second of these three levels, particularly the early detection of periodontal disease in adolescents through public health screening. As far as we are aware no public health service operates a systematic programme of screening for periodontal disease. Nevertheless, this should not prevent the examination and consideration of such a possibility.

The review therefore has four broad aims:

1. To review some of the general principles of public health screening.
2. To provide an account of research conducted by the Dental Health Unit of the University of Manchester during the early 1970s on the prevalence of early periodontal disease in teenagers and on the possibility of developing a screening test to detect such subjects.
3. To review and discuss some of the limitations and criticisms of that early work.
4. To provide a preliminary account of further work recently completed which attempts to answer some of those criticisms.

General Principles of Screening for Disease

A screening test may be defined as a simple test to select a group of subjects who would benefit from more detailed examination and diagnosis. The aims of screening are first to detect disease at an earlier stage than that at which a subject would normally present for treatment, and second to provide treatment that would alter, for the better, the natural history of the disease. Clearly, the screening examination should be acceptable to those on whom it is conducted and the benefits of screening should outweigh the costs of conducting the programme. There is however a further principle which is less immediately obvious. Any screening examination, indeed any diagnostic examination, will result in errors and these errors will be of two types. Firstly, the screening test may classify as 'healthy', subjects who do in fact have the disease and, secondly, the test may mistakenly classify as 'diseased', subjects who are in fact healthy. The proportion or percentage of truly diseased subjects correctly identified by the test is defined as the sensitivity of the test, while the proportion of truly nondiseased subjects correctly identified is defined as the specificity of the test. The ideal test should have high sensitivity and high specificity although, as will be discussed, these attributes can often be gained only at the expense of the other.

Loss of Attachment in 15-Year-Old Children

In 1973 an epidemiological study was conducted on the prevalence of early loss of attachment in all 15-year-old children attending schools in one administrative area close to Manchester. This study was part of a wider study aimed at developing the methodology of treatment need studies, and the results of the study have been published elsewhere.[2, 4, 5] The basic premise underlying these studies was that gingivitis, which is almost universally present in British teenagers, could not be considered as indicating a treatment need. Rather, priority for treatment should be given to those subjects in whom disease was progressing beyond gingivitis to the early breakdown of the periodontal supporting tissues. Briefly, loss of attachment was measured using a standardised periodontal probe on the mesiobuccal aspects of first permanent molars and on the distobuccal aspects of permanent incisors. The prevalence of loss of attachment was surprisingly high, with 46% of the subjects having loss of attachment of at least 1 mm and 11% having loss of attachment of at least 2 mm on at least one tooth. Children of West-Indian or Indo-Pakistani origin seemed particularly susceptible, as did children of lower academic attainment.

The measurement of loss of attachment is not a simple procedure and would not be suitable as a screening procedure for large groups of children. We examined, therefore, whether simpler criteria such as the presence of obvious plaque, gingival

bleeding or subgingival calculus, could predict the presence of loss of attachment. A summary of the findings are presented in Table 16.1. It was decided, quite arbitrarily, that the 167 subjects with loss of attachment of at least 1 mm on at least two teeth would be considered diseased, while the rest would be considered healthy.

It is clear from Table 16.1 that a screening test based on the presence of plaque or gingival bleeding would correctly identify most of the children with loss of attachment (sensitivity = 83.2% and 91.6% respectively). However, it is also clear that because of the low values for specificity (25.7% and 30.5% respectively) that many subjects would be incorrectly classified as diseased. In contrast, although subgingival calculus had a slightly lower value for sensitivity 76.6%, the value for specificity 69.5% was considerably higher. A screening test based on subgingival calculus would therefore identify a relatively small group of children, a high proportion of whom would actually have loss of attachment.

Limitations of this Study

It is clear that there are limitations in the study reported and these might broadly be considered as follows:

1. The accuracy with which the base of the periodontal pocket could be identified, when probing for loss of attachment, was not known.
2. The study was cross-sectional in design and no evidence was presented that the levels of loss of attachment reported were pathological changes rather than simple developmental abnormalities that had been present throughout.
3. By 15 years of age many children in Britain would be due to leave school and would not therefore be eligible for a

Table 16.1 The sensitivity and specificity of three predictors of the presence of loss of attachment in 622 subjects aged 15 years.

Loss of attachment	Positive[1] (Number of subjects) 167		Negative (Number of subjects) 455	
Predictors	Positives correctly predicted		Negatives correctly predicted	
	Number	% (Sensitivity)	Number	% (Specificity)
Plaque	139	83.2	117	25.7
Gingival bleeding	153	91.6	139	30.5
Subgingival calculus	128	76.6	316	69.5

[1] A subject was deemed positive if he/she had loss of attachment of at least 1 mm on at least two teeth at age 15 years.

periodontal treatment programme in the public health service, even if such a programme existed.

4. It would seem more sensible to identify subjects at risk to loss of attachment rather than to await its onset.
5. The extent to which treatment could prevent or retard the progression of loss of attachment was not known, and it was therefore difficult to justify a screening programme.

In an attempt to answer at least some of these criticisms, a further longitudinal study of loss of attachment in teenage subjects was conducted.

Longitudinal Study on the Progression of Loss of Attachment in Teenage Subjects

As a preliminary to this study, a series of investigations were undertaken to establish the validity of loss of attachment as a measure of the early breakdown of the periodontal supporting tissues, which

supplemented others, had appeared in the literature between 1974 and 1980.[7] Basically, the method followed was to measure loss of attachment on teeth scheduled for extraction then, having extracted the tooth, to stain the periodontal fibres attached to the root surface with some appropriate laboratory stain and remeasure loss of attachment by direct observation. The results are summarized in Table 16.2, where it can be seen that there is a close agreement between the clinical and laboratory measurements of loss of attachment. A number of studies[7] have suggested that in the presence of gingivitis the probe may enter the connective tissues and over-estimate the loss of attachment. Our own studies support this contention, but it is important to recognize that at the level of measurement used in epidemiological studies (i.e. to the nearest whole mm) these over- or under-estimates of attachment loss are not clinically significant.

The next stage was to conduct a 2 year longitudinal study of loss of attachment in 229 teenage children, starting at age 14 years through to age 16 years. This study

Table 16.2 Comparison of clinical and laboratory measures of loss of attachment on the mesio – buccal surface of 71 teeth.

Clinical loss of attachment	Number of surfaces	Laboratory loss of attachment		% correct
		Absent (0 mm)	Present (1 – 3 mm)	
Absent (0 mm)	43	41	2	95
Present (1 – 3 mm)	28	1	27	96

Table 16.3 The sensitivity and specificity of four baseline predictors of the development of loss of attachment over a subsequent 2 year period in 229 subjects aged 14 years at baseline.

Loss of attachment over 2 year period	Positive[1] (Number of subjects) 53		Negative (Number of subjects) 176	
Baseline Predictor	Positives correctly predicted		Negatives correctly predicted	
	Number	% (Sensitivity)	Number	% (Specificity)
Unequivocal colour change in gingivae	28	52.80	125	71.02
Gingival bleeding	39	73.60	63	35.80
Plaque	44	83.00	70	39.80
Subgingival calculus	22	41.50	155	88.10

[1] A subject was deemed positive if he/she developed loss of attachment of at least 1 mm on at least two teeth over the 2 years of the study.

has recently been completed. At the beginning, 10 subjects (4%) had loss of attachment of at least 1 mm on at least 1 tooth, while 2 years later the prevalence had increased to 39%. In Table 16.3 the ability of baseline measures of plaque, gingival bleeding, unequivocal colour change and subgingival calculus to predict subsequent loss of attachment, which developed over the 2 years of the study, is considered. As in the earlier study, gingival bleeding and plaque provide high values for sensitivity, with most subjects, who developed loss of attachment over the course of the study, having gingival bleeding and obvious supragingival plaque at baseline. However, the low values for specificity indicate that many other subjects with gingival bleeding and plaque at baseline did *not* develop loss of attachment. In contrast, a screening test based on subgingival calculus would have high specificity and low sensitivity. The test would identify only a small group of subjects, many of whom would subsequently develop loss of attachment. However, because of the low value for sensitivity, the test would also miss some subjects who subsequently developed loss of attachment. Unequivocal colour change, which was not measured in the earlier cross-sectional study, provides intermediate values for both sensitivity and specificity. In summary, therefore, a highly sensitive test will ensure that very few cases are missed, and a highly specific test will ensure that the treatment programme will not be overwhelmed by subjects who are not at risk to loss of attachment. The balance to be struck between those two conflicting objectives would obviously be a public health decision rather than a statistical one.[5]

Discussion

The data presented from the recent longitudinal study go a considerable way to answering four of the five criticisms listed earlier. However, there remains the key problem of whether effective treatment can be provided for those subjects identified at 14 years of age to be at risk to loss of attachment. This is not simply a matter of whether a treatment procedure is available, because clearly there are commonly available methods of treating subjects with obvious plaque, gingival bleeding and subgingival calculus deposits. Rather, the question is how *effective* is that treatment. The dilemma has been posed very clearly by *Sheiham*,[8] who explains the difference between screening where the dentist is actively seeking out patients for treatment, and the more usual situation where the initiative is left to the patients themselves. In the latter case the dentist must provide treatment to the best of his ability, according to current knowledge, even if that knowledge is deficient; in the case of screening, however, the dentist must assure himself that *effective treatment* is available before undertaking a screening programme, and if he cannot so assure himself he should not undertake screening. In other words, health authorities should not create a demand for treatments not known to be effective.

To what extent, then, are current treatment regimes effective and how should effectiveness be defined? *Sheiham*[8] has suggested that the effectiveness of periodontal therapy should be evaluated in terms of its ability to prevent tooth loss from periodontal disease, arguing that the total prevention of attachment loss is not necessary, but rather that the rate of attachment loss should be sufficiently slow to ensure that subjects retain adequate periodontal support for their lifetimes. However, this criterion poses considerable problems to the public health dentist who is considering a programme to improve the periodontal health of children and teenagers in his target population. If the criterion for effectiveness is that the programme should be shown to reduce tooth loss from periodontal disease, then clinical trials of unrealistic length would be required. It is therefore necessary to determine more realistic subgoals. In Britain it was determined in 1964 that the objectives of the school dental service would include ensuring that children should leave school free of dental disease and dental irregularity.[6] In the case of periodontal health it would not seem unreasonable to interpret that objective as 'leaving school with no teeth affected by loss of attachment'. A similar proposal was made by a recent WHO Workshop.[9]

If this proposal is accepted, then the question concerning effectiveness can be redefined – to what extent can treatment prevent the onset of loss of attachment by the age of 16 years? On presently avail-

215

able evidence it should be possible to prevent loss of attachment in young adults,[1] but whether such a programme would be effective, acceptable and economic in teenagers is not known. However, we have satisfied ourselves that a longitudinal study on loss of attachment in teenage children is not difficult to conduct, and therefore answers concerning the acceptability and cost-effectiveness of treatment programmes for teenage children at high risk to periodontal disease could be provided within 3 to 4 years.

References

1. *Axelsson P.* and *Lindhe J.*
   Effect of controlled oral hygiene procedures on caries and periodontal disease in adults: results after six years. J. Clin. Periodontol., 1981, 8: 239–248.

2. *Bowden D. E. J., Davies R. M., Holloway P. J., Lennon M. A.* and *Rugg-Gunn A. J.*
   A treatment need survey of a 15-year-old population. Brit. Dent. J., 1973, 134: 375–379.

3. *Gjermo P*
   Establishment of priorities in periodontal care. In Efficacy of Treatment procedures in Periodontics. (Shanley, D., ed.) Quintessence, Chicago, 1980, pp. 317–324.

4. *Lennon M. A.* and *Davies R. M.*
   Prevalence and distribution of alveolar bone loss in a population of 15-year-old schoolchildren. J. Clin. Periodontol., 1974, 1: 175–182.

5. *Lennon M. A.* and *Davies R. M.*
   A method for defining the level of periodontal treatment need in a population of 15-year-old schoolchildren. Community Dent. Oral Epidemiol., 1975, 3: 244–249.

6. *Lennon M. A.*
   The organisation of dental services in the United Kingdom. In Dental Public Health: An Introduction to Community Dental Health. 2nd edn (G. L. Slack, ed.) J. Wright, Bristol 1981.

7. *Listgarten M. A.*
   Periodontal probing: what does it mean? J. Clin. Periodontol., 1980, 7: 165–176.

8. *Sheiham A.*
   Screening for periodontal disease. J. Clin. Periodontol., 1978, 5: 237–245.

9. *World Health Organisation.*
   A review of current recommendations for the organisation and administration of community oral health services in Northern and Western Europe. WHO Regional Office, Copenhagen 1983.

17. Current Status of Nonsurgical and Surgical Periodontal Treatment

Niklaus P. Lang

Nonsurgical Periodontal Treatment

In 1882, *Riggs* emphasized the significance of tooth scaling for the treatment and prevention of periodontal disease. In his lecture on the so-called 'pyorrhea alveolaris' he advocated the most simple concept for conservative periodontal therapy: 'When you find a tooth with the characteristic concentration of tartar upon it, the first principle of surgery demands that you clean that tooth thoroughly . . . and in 3 days you will notice a marked improvement for the better'.[45] Although similar thoughts have been expressed in ancient cultures more than 1000 years ago, it was not until approximately 20 years ago that the bacterial aetiology of gingivitis and destructive periodontitis was convincingly established on the basis of epidemiological[4, 29] and clinical experimental studies.[28] Only a few years ago, controlled clinical trials in man have documented[5] that advanced periodontal disease and dental caries may be arrested by complete plaque control. In addition, during the last decade, dog experiments have shown that destructive periodontal disease can be prevented by mechanical plaque control in otherwise susceptible animals.[24, 30]
In the view of this accumulated knowledge, it is obvious that effective periodontal therapy is based on the skillful performance of both the patient and the dentist.

It is the patient's responsibility to make an effort in maintaining clean teeth and, consequently, healthy gingival tissues by adequate oral hygiene procedures, the goal of which must be the continuous and complete mechanical removal of bacterial plaque. On the other hand, it is the responsibility of the professional to competently motivate and instruct the patient and to eliminate all soft and hard deposits on the tooth surfaces at regular intervals. The goal of these procedures is the elimination of bacterial irritants on and within the surfaces of the teeth in order to provide biological acceptable smooth and clean surfaces to which healing of the gingival and periodontal tissues can take place predictably.[43]
Nonsurgical periodontal therapy, therefore, consists of patient motivation, instruction in oral hygiene procedures and thorough scaling and root planing of the teeth.

Motivation and Instruction in Oral Hygiene

Since a direct cause and effect relationship has been established between bacterial plaque and gingivitis,[28] the routine and complete removal of these deposits must represent the most important challenge for successful periodontal therapy and prevention of future loss of attachment. As shown by *Cumming* and *Löe*,[12] each patient performs oral hygiene procedures in a specific pattern. If subjects are evaluated at multiple examinations according to their plaque indices, it is evident that similar tooth surfaces consistently remain uncleaned or cleaned irrespective of the quality of performance.

Not only people with poor oral hygiene, but also those with relatively good oral hygiene, leave substantial amounts of plaque on, for example the lower lingual and the interproximal surfaces of the teeth.[12] In order to break the pattern of oral hygiene, multiple plaque assessments are indicated during hygienic phase.[22]

It has also been established that, for maintenance of periodontal health, complete plaque control has to be performed only every 24–48 hours.[21] When volunteers performed supervised and complete oral hygiene procedures at different intervals, different amounts of plaque deposits were seen in the different groups. However, only if the oral hygiene interval exceeded 48 hours did gingivitis develop during the 6 week experimental period. These findings clearly indicated that one daily but complete plaque removal may be more efficient for a good prognosis than, for example, five daily oral hygiene procedures performed in an incomplete and superficial manner.[21]

Results of Clinical Trials

In order to substantiate the hypothesis that continous and complete plaque removal will prevent dental plaque diseases such as tooth decay and chronic periodontitis, *Axelsson* and *Lindhe*[5] described a maintenance care programme which involved professional prophylaxis procedures once every 2–3 months in order to supplement a successful plaque control programme of patients with advanced

periodontal disease. This meticulous programme in oral hygiene, together with the continous reinforcement at the recall visits, was successful in completely preventing the recurrence of periodontitis after it had been treated. Furthermore, and perhaps even more surprising, dental caries was practically eliminated by this sustained high standard of oral hygiene. Even after an observation period of 6 years, not more than 2% of the gingival units bled on gentle probing. Consequently, very shallow pockets (mean 1.6 mm) were maintained and no probing attachment was lost during the entire period of 6 years. In contrast, pockets tended to recur in the control group concomittantly with more sites of gingival units which bled on probing (up to 45%). Furthermore, the control group lost between 0.13 and 0.26 mm of probing attachment per year. Since practically no new or recurrent carious lesions developed in over 300 patients during the observation period, it can be concluded that, indeed, caries and periodontal diseases may effectively be prevented by sustained high standards of oral hygiene.[5]

Animal experiments have also demonstrated that following an initial scaling and root planing, periodontal attachment levels can be maintained by oral hygiene measures only.[30] Repeated scaling did not influence the maintenance of the probing attachment level when bacterial plaque was continously removed for a period of up to 3 years.

Consequently, a high standard of oral hygiene either achieved by the patient's own performance, or by repeated professional care, is an absolute prerequisite for periodontal therapy, be it conservative or surgical in nature. For any further discussion of the conservative treatment it will, therefore, be assumed that these principles enjoy unrestricted validity.

Scaling and Root Planing

The terms 'scaling' and 'root planing' are traditionally used to indicate a complete removal of calcified hard deposits on the teeth and thus creating a smooth and glass-hard surface[50] with the aim to make the tooth biologically acceptable to the soft tissues.[43]

The beneficial effects of subgingival calculus removal on gingival health, pocket depth and attachment levels have been documented in numerous clinical[2, 15, 17, 44] and histological reports.[3, 16, 33, 55, 56, 57] Waerhaug[56] observed calculus on the root surface surrounded by degenerated epithelial cells and epithelial proliferation into the connective tissue, as well as apical migration on the junctional epithelium concommittantly with inflammatory cells close to the bottom of the periodontal pockets. However, as soon as the calculus was removed, healing took place and only minor inflammatory cell aggregates and minimal epithelial proliferation was noted closely associated with residual calculus deposits. Although the rationale for scaling seems to be accepted by general practitioners as well as researchers, the rationale for deliberately root planing the tooth surfaces is still under dispute. It is evident that rough tooth surfaces will enhance plaque formation. In the subgingival area, this might be of crucial significance.[57] Root planing has also been advocated for the elimination of contaminated root cementum, hereby removing bacterial endotoxins from roots of periodontally involved teeth.[17] The presence of cementum-bound lipopolysaccharide endotoxins in areas of periodontal pockets has been indicated in studies by *Aleo et al.*[1] However, it is not known how deep the toxin will penetrate and, hence, how much of the tooth substance will have to be removed. Without doubt root planing will enhance the chance of complete removal of calculus,[50] the most significant retaining factor for subgingival bacterial plaque.

Therefore, from a clinical point of view, the tactile test of root surface smoothness represents a crude but probably effective way to ensure complete elimination of hard deposits, although minute pieces may persist following instrumentation in scratches and grooves which are undetectable by sense of touch.[35, 58]

Healing following scaling and root planing

Immediately following scaling and root planing the epithelial attachment is severed and the junctional and crevicular epithelium partially removed. There is a danger that, with severe inflammation, scaling will extend apically to the bottom of the epithelial attachment and tear healthy connective tissue fibres. In 4 to 5 days, a new long epithelial attachment may regenerate in the bottom part of the crevice. However, complete healing normally occurs in 1 to 2 weeks, depending on the severity of inflammation and the depth of the periodontal pocket.[54]

Residual rete pegs in the crevice wall after scaling appear to undergo involution[43] and a normal epithelial attachment will form. As indicated, the clinical healing process following scaling and root planing depends much on the resolution of gingivitis following adequate plaque control.

Bacteriological aspects of scaling and root planing

It has recently been reported[32, 51] that the composition of the subgingival microbial flora is completely altered by even single scaling and root planing procedures. The recolonization of the subgingival flora with proportions of organisms characteristic for periodontal pockets may vary from 42 days[32] to 3–4 months.[51] Using darkfield microscopy, *Listgarten, Lindhe & Helldèn*[27] also monitored the composition of the subgingival microflora undergoing treatment. Very clearly, certain shifts in the microbial flora took place following mechanical debridement or antibiotic therapy. Microbial alterations were induced by mechanical debridement 2–8 weeks following the last intervention and were still detectable after 25 weeks.

From these microbiological data it might be speculated that the periodic recall prophylaxis every 3–4 months may prevent the reestablishment of a periodontopathic flora. These thoughts are further substantiated by microbiological data from an animal experiment in which, by a single course of scaling and root planing followed by controlled oral hygiene, attachment levels were maintained during a period of 3 years.[53]

Animal Experiments

For many years, different surgical treatment modalities have been accepted in periodontal therapy. Since it is considered unethical to deny accepted treatment procedures, scaling and root planing alone have not been evaluated in human clinical trials for many years. For this reason, an animal experiment was performed for 3 years in beagle dogs,[31] in which the effect of conservative periodontal therapy was to be studied in conjunction with or without controlled oral hygiene procedure. In this study, 8 beagle dogs with moderate naturally developed periodontitis were assigned to either a test or control group. The test group (4 dogs) received a thorough scaling and root planing at the start of the experiment. Thereafter, the dogs were subjected to daily toothbrushing and a rubber cup prophylaxis every 2 weeks. The control animals were not subjected to any oral hygiene procedures. Two quadrants diagonally opposed in each test and control animals were scaled and root planed every 6 months.

The dogs of the test group showed an in-

creased and maintained clinical attachment throughout the study. Initial scaling and root planing, followed by oral hygiene, reduced probing depth significantly, a result which was maintained over the 3 year period. Repeated scaling did not influence the maintenance of the achieved results in the test group. However, the control animals continued to loose clinical attachment and probing depth increased during the study. In this group, i.e. without oral hygiene, repeated scaling every 6 months resulted in loss of clinical attachment at a rate which was clearly retarded. This animal study provided encouraging findings that nonsurgical periodontal therapy, in conjunction with oral hygiene, may maintain periodontal clinical attachment levels in moderate periodontitis cases. However, in the absence of oral hygiene, nonsurgical periodontal therapy may only significantly retard the progression of destructive periodontitis, most likely by altering the subgingival microenvironment at regular intervals[13].

Human Clinical Trials of Short Duration

In the 1960s and 1970s most human clinical trials were performed to evaluate different surgical treatment modalities for periodontal therapy.[10, 19, 20, 31, 37, 38, 40, 41, 47, 48, 49, 59, 60, 61, 62] Only one of these studies[59] has compared nonsurgical periodontal therapy to conventional gingivectomies over 48 weeks. Slight reductions in probing depth and maintenance of clinical attachment levels were reported following scaling and root planing only, although pocket reduction was smaller than when gingivectomies were performed.[59]

However, one recent study carefully evaluated the beneficial effects of hygienic phase.[31] The initial periodontal status in 90 patients with moderate to advanced periodontitis was compared with the clinical parameters one month following completion of a hygienic phase, which included patient motivation, instruction in oral hygiene and thorough scaling and root planing. Obviously, plaque, calculus and gingivitis were reduced significantly, although not absolutely perfect plaque scores had been obtained. However, the surprising findings indicated there was a mean pocket reduction of approximately 1 mm in pockets which originally presented with 4–6 mm probing depth and 2 mm reduction in pockets with an initial probing depth of 7–12 mm. About half of the reduction was due to resolution of gingival oedema, resulting in recession of the free gingival margin. The other half was due to gain of clinical attachment from the bottom of the pockets. Similar favourable results have been reported by several authors.[15, 55]

Longterm Clinical Trials

As mentioned, the early epidemiological studies of *Lövdal et al*[29] had already demonstrated the longterm beneficial effect of scaling and root planing, combined with oral hygiene procedures.

When the group at the University of Michigan found that scaling and root planing, in conjunction with oral hygiene, could maintain attachment levels over 3 years in beagle dogs,[30] they continued their longitudinal study beyond the observation period of the hygienic phase[31] and recently presented a 2 year follow-up report.[14] The 90 patients received four different treatment modalities in each of the four quadrants of the dentition. While three treatment procedures included surgical intervention, the fourth quadrant received scaling and root planing only. The results indicated that, in sulci which were 1–3 mm deep, a slight reduction in probing depth occurred with all the procedures including scaling and root planing only. However, this group of sulci slightly

lost attachment over the 2 years, with all the treatment modalities performed. In pockets, which initially scored 4–6 mm, the main pocket reduction occurred after hygienic phase but the pockets were further reduced by surgical therapy. However, this pocket reduction had no additional beneficial effect on the maintenance of the clinical attachment level which, in this group of pockets, was best maintained following nonsurgical therapy only. For deep pockets of 7 mm or more, pocket reduction was achieved by the hygienic phase and by the surgical procedures. But again, this pocket reduction did not significantly influence the maintenance of the level of the gained clinical attachment following hygienic phase.[14]

Another report presented similar longterm results in a well organized clinical trial.[34] In this study, 17 patients received modified Widman flap procedures, or scaling and root planing only in a split mouth design. The study showed that, although there was less pocket reduction with scaling and root planing alone, clinical attachment was gained and maintained equally well over 6½ years with nonsurgical therapy as when additional flaps were performed. In sulci of 1–3 mm depth, and in pockets 4–6 mm in size, significantly more clinical attachment was obtained with the nonsurgical therapy.[34]

The most recent report of all confirming these longitudinal studies originates from the University of Gothenburg.[25] In this trial, 15 patients with advanced periodontal disease were subjected to periodontal therapy, utilizing a split mouth design. Either nonsurgical subgingival debridement was performed in conjunction with a modified Widman flap, or therapy was restricted to scaling and root planing only. Again, it was concluded that scaling and root planing alone were almost equally effective as their application in combination with surgical periodontal therapy in establishing clinically healthy gingivae and in preventing further loss of attachment. However, sites with periodontal surgery and initial probing depth of 7 mm or more showed significant gain of clinical attachment. Loss of clinical attachment did not occur in sites treated nonsurgically. Again, in 4–6 mm deep pockets, nonsurgical therapy was equally effective in maintaining clinical attachment levels as therapy, including flap procedures, despite the fact that the surgical procedures were slightly more effective in reducing probing depth. Furthermore, this study has demonstrated that pocket reduction by surgical flap procedures was significantly larger in single-rooted than in multirooted teeth. However, when scaling and root planing was performed alone, there was no statistical significance between the pocket reduction in single or multirooted teeth. This may present some limitations to nonsurgical procedures when deep periodontal pockets are to be reduced in multirooted teeth. It has also been demonstrated that these teeth often present with involved furcations in which access for root planing is poor.[11, 16] Teeth with furcation involvements are difficult to treat and were found to be the most frequently lost teeth in the Michigan longitudinal study.[20] Obviously, scaling and root planing are difficult treatment procedures and may take not only skilful operators but also extended time for therapy.[25] The deeper the periodontal pockets the greater is the chance that calculus deposits may be left on the root surface.[35] It would seem logical to suggest that nonsurgical treatment for advanced periodontal disease may be limited by both access to the full extent of a lesion as well as by the operator's experience and skill.

This has to be kept in mind when the last series of clinical studies by *Badersten, Nilvéus* and *Egelberg*[7, 8, 9] are to be evaluated. The incisors, cuspids and bicuspids of 15 patients were only treated with nonsurgical procedures. Using a split mouth design, one half of the dentition was instrumented with hand instruments and the other half with ultrasonic instruments. Of the original 528 pockets, 184 were 5 mm or more in the beginning of this first study.[7] Only 31 presented with such depths following hygienic phase. Similar results of up to 80% reductions in the number of deep pockets[8] documented the crucial role of the hygienic phase of periodontal therapy. Also this group of researchers were able to maintain such favourable results over a period of 1½ to 2 years.

However, it has to be kept in mind that, in all studies mentioned in this review, good oral hygiene procedures and regular scaling of accumulated hard deposits were assured by recall visits at various intervals of 3–6 months. It has clearly been demonstrated that successful pocket reduction and gained levels of clinical attachment, irrespective of the treatment modalities which led to the clinical success, can only be maintained by well organized recall systems.[6] If patients are left by themselves, the great majority will continue to lose periodontal attachment as a result of recurrent periodontitis.[5, 6, 18]

Surgical Periodontal Treatment

For many decades periodontal surgical procedures have been an integral part of periodontal therapy and a great variety of procedures have been advocated, each with a different rationale. Recently, *Barrington*[10] has presented a comprehensive review of periodontal surgical procedures. Therefore, only principle aspects will be discussed here emphasizing the comparisons of different procedures on the basis of well-controlled longitudinal clinical trials.

Basically, periodontal surgery may be divided into five different categories:

1. Subgingival curettage.
2. Gingivectomy or flap surgery for pocket elimination.

3. Treatment of osseous defects.
4. Flap surgery for reattachment.
5. Mucogingival surgical procedures.

Subgingival curettage

This procedure aims at the complete and deliberate removal of the soft tissue lining of a periodontal pocket. While the procedure has been described as an isolated surgical intervention following scaling and root planing,[37] it is evident that this procedure is also combined with the latter in clinical practice. On the other hand, it is clear that scaling and root planing alone may also remove parts of the soft tissue lining of the periodontal pocket. Hence, the assessment of efficacy of removing the soft tissue pocket lining as an isolated procedure becomes difficult.

Gingivectomy or flap surgery for pocket elimination

The goal of these procedures is to eliminate pockets by removing soft tissue and/or recontouring it in order to obtain gingival tissues with a healthy sulcus not exceeding 3 mm in depth. However, if periodontal lesions have progressed apically into the supporting bone, these goals have to be reached by removing and/or recontouring osseous tissue. Generally, pocket elimination is achieved by gingivectomies if the periodontal lesions are characterized by horizontal bone loss and not extending apically to the mucogingival junction. In the instance of infrabony lesions and pockets extending apically to the mucogingival junction, mucoperiosteal flaps with apical repositioning are performed.

Treatment of osseous defects

Osseous surgery has been advocated in combination with apically repositioned flaps. While osseous defects may be eliminated, using either ostectomy or osteoplasty to resect or recontour alveolar bone adjacent to the osseous defects, attempts have been made to replace lost alveolar bone in these defects with different grafting procedures. Since well-controlled longterm results are not available for any of these procedures, they cannot be advocated as routine practice. The main question is whether grafting materials are able to induce bone formation, connective tissue fibre attachment and cementogenesis, or whether they act more like a scaffold in the healing of an osseous defect.

Flap surgery for reattachment

The goal of these procedures is to create optimal conditions for reattachment and, if possible, new attachment. These interventions include the modified Widman flap,[39] the excisional new attachment procedure (ENAP),[60] open flap curettage[52] and other 'replaced' flaps. The main feature is the minimal excision of gingival tissues, the minimal extent of flap reflection, the close adaptation of the tissues and the suturing near the presurgical position of the gingival margin. Since all of these procedures provide open access to the root surfaces, they have also been termed 'access flaps'.[46]

Mucogingival surgical procedures

A great variety of surgical procedures have been described to correct mucogingival problems, deficiencies and deformities. However, the indications for these procedures have been disputed in recent years. Longterm well controlled studies are in process, but not enough conclusive evidence has been presented as to their value. A thorough discussion on the topic is beyond the limit of this review but, from a public health point of view, it may be stated that surgical procedures to correct the width of keratinized gingiva and/ or to eliminate frenum pull are of a very minor importance.

Results from Clinical Trials

Twenty years ago, the indications and the selection of certain periodontal surgical interventions were based on clinical judgment and the personal preference of the operator, rather than on scientific evidence. In 1961, the first controlled longitudinal study on the efficacy of the accepted treatment procedures of that time was started at the University of Michigan. The first report of the pioneer work of *Ramfjord* and his *co-workers*[37] appeared in 1968 and compared clinical data on surgical pocket elimination procedures with subgingival curettage. Subsequently, numerous longitudinal studies of different length have been presented by the same group of authors[14, 19, 20, 31, 38, 40, 41, 43] and by other investigators.[5, 6, 7, 8, 9, 13, 25, 27, 34, 36, 47, 48, 59, 60, 61, 62] These studies included other categories of periodontal surgery such as modified Widman flaps, ENAP, different flaps with and without osseous resection. However, only recently all the surgical procedures were evaluated against the nonsurgical periodontal treatment[5, 7, 8, 9, 14, 25, 31, 34] because periodontal surgery was an accepted part of periodontal therapy. Since it is considered unethical to deny accepted treatment procedures to patients, these studies had to be done in animal experiments[23, 30] prior to human trials.

It has to be realized that major differences exist among the different studies. These include differences in initial disease severity and methodological design, such as split-mouth versus group design, and differences in clinical parameters for evaluation. Also, the degree of plaque control

and, even more important, different recall intervals may account for slight variations in the results obtained. Most recently, a clear overview of the different studies mentioned has been presented.[46] Therefore, this review will present only the generally accepted longitudinal concepts based on the numerous different longitudinal studies emphasizing clinical periodontal attachment levels and probing depths.

Animal Experiments

A 3-year longitudinal study in Beagle dogs[23] evaluated the therapeutic effects of periodontal surgery on clinical attachment levels and probing depths and compared them with those of nonsurgical periodontal therapy. The following treatments were compared with each other in a quadrant design:

1. Subgingival curettage.
2. Modified Widman flap.
3. Apically repositioned flap and bone surgery for pocket elimination.
4. Scaling and root planing as a control.

Daily toothbrushing and rubber cup and pumice prophylaxes assured optimal plaque control throughout the 3 years. The postsurgical results at one month showed increased clinical attachment levels which were maintained for the 3-year period following any of the surgical interventions. Also, the reduced probing depths were maintained throughout the experimental period. In advanced periodontitis, scaling and root planing alone were not able to maintain the clinical attachment levels and the reduced probing depths gained initially. However, clinical attachment was still at a more coronal level after 3 years than it was initially. This study has demonstrated that more conservative approaches to the treatment of periodontal disease, such as subgingival curettage and modified Widman flap surgery, may be as effective in maintaining clinical attachment levels as elaborate surgical procedures involving osteotectomy.

Human Clinical Trials of Short Duration

Short-term studies of 4–6 months[52, 62] used a split-mouth design to evaluate either subgingival curettage and/or apically repositioned flaps with access flaps. All the procedures were essentially equally effective in reducing pockets. While subgingival curettage gained some clinical attachment, the flap procedures were associated with a slight initial loss. This loss was more pronounced when osseous surgery was performed. Similar results were obtained in clinical trials of 2 years duration.[14, 37, 40, 47, 48] These reports presented results which were generated by two completely different studies at the University of Michigan[14, 37, 40] and the University of Gothenburg.[47, 48] While the former used a split-mouth design and recall intervals of 3 months, the latter presented a group approach and applied the professional tooth cleaning system[5] in recall visits every 2 weeks for optimal plaque control. Yet, similar results were obtained for all the procedures. Pocket reduction was greater with access flaps and pocket reduction surgery than with subgingival curettage. Some gain of clinical attachment was noted with subgingival curettage and access flaps, while loss of clinical attachment was consistently found associated with pocket elimination procedures. On the basis of these studies it is apparent that the gain and maintenance of clinical attachment is not necessarily related to the reduction in probing depth.

Longterm Clinical Trials

The observations that osseous surgery may have no advantage in maintaining longterm attachment levels was later documented in several well-controlled clinical trials of long duration.[19, 20, 34, 36, 40, 42, 61] It is evident that subgingival curettage, access flaps and pocket elimination surgery are effective in reducing probing depths, irrespective of the procedures performed. However, clinical attachment levels were best increased with subgingival curettage, modified Widman flap and ENAP. However, the differences in the values measured are so small that they probably lack clinical relevance, even though they are statistically significant. A few studies[14, 19, 34, 40] can be compared with each other on the basis of presurgical disease severity.[46] It is evident that all the surgical procedures will result in a slight loss of clinical attachment of up to 1 mm if sulci of 1–3 mm probing depths are incorporated in the treatment. However, moderate periodontal pockets of 4–6 mm probing depths before treatment will demonstrate slightly increased clinical attachment levels irrespective of the surgical procedures carried out. The greatest gain of clinical attachment levels for all the procedures was noted in advanced periodontitis with pretreatment probing depths of 7–12 mm. In those deep pockets the access flaps seemed to be the most predictable procedures over the years.[19, 20] It is also evident, especially from the studies of the University of Michigan[14, 19] and the University of Gothenburg,[48, 49] that access flap procedures which did not include osseous resection or recontouring are at least as effective as flap procedures including bone surgery. Interproximal healing of bony defects was identical in two studies[47, 52] of up to 2 years observation. Also, in the very deep periodontal pockets of the Michigan longitudinal study,[19] the healing of osseous defects was identical whether bone resection had been performed or not.

Conclusion

In conclusion, numerous longitudinal studies in the last 2 decades have been performed with different study designs and different postsurgical maintenance programmes. Although the inherent difficulties of clinical research have to be considered, a few conclusions may be drawn which are unanimously accepted by most clinical scientists:

1. Gain or loss of clinical periodontal attachment is not primarily dependent on any particular type of periodontal surgery.
2. With all procedures employed, clinical attachment is slightly lost in sulci of initial probing depth of 1–3 mm.
3. In moderate periodontitis of 4–6 mm probing depth clinical attachment levels are maintained with all procedures.
4. In advanced periodontitis of 7–12 mm probing depth clinical attachment may be gained with all procedures.
5. Postsurgical clinical attachment levels are not related to the degree of the reduction in probing depth.
6. Osseous surgery is not a necessary requirement for reducing probing depths or maintaining clinical attachment.
7. The deliberate removal of the soft tissue lining of periodontal pockets by subgingival curettage is not an advantageous procedure over scaling and root planing alone.
8. Results obtained by periodontal surgical procedures can be maintained over many years provided that postsurgical maintenance care is assured.

Significance for clinical practice

There is a great number of well-designed and controlled clinical trials which clearly document that nonsurgical periodontal therapy including patient motivation, instruction in oral hygiene and thorough scaling and root planing is a feasible method for treating moderate chronic destructive periodontal disease, provided that the patient's performance can be supervised at regular maintenance intervals. There is also increasing evidence that this nonsurgical approach will be successful in effectively treating deep periodontal pockets and maintaining clinical attachment levels. To what extent nonsurgical treatment will be superior to surgical interventions has not yet been conclusively established. Efforts have been made to point out 'critical probing depth' for different treatment modalities[19, 26] in order to provide the clinician with more clear-cut information for treatment planning. It appears from the longitudinal studies that the 'critical probing depth', at which nonsurgical procedures would provide more favourable healing than flap procedures, may be greater than previously considered.[19, 26] Therefore, moderate periodontal pockets of initially 4–7 mm depth should first be subjected to careful nonsurgical periodontal therapy before the indications for a surgical intervention is assigned.[7, 8] However, it has to be remembered, that the main problem with scaling and root planing is the difficulty in gaining access to root surfaces in teeth with furcation involvement and deep periodontal lesions. Successful nonsurgical therapy might in these instances require more time and manpower than if those procedures are performed in conjunction with periodontal surgery.

Therefore, the treatment of deep periodontal pockets may still be performed by surgical intervention. Flaps for access have been shown to be the most predictable procedures with respect to maintaining or gaining clinical attachment. Furthermore, osseous resection is not a required procedure to obtain optimal healing of angular bone resorption and osseous defects. The postsurgical maintenance programme with recall visit intervals not exceeding 3–4 months may be a prerequisite for the successful maintenance of the treatment result obtained by nonsurgical or surgical periodontal therapy.

References

1. *Aleo J. J., Renzis F. A., Farber P. A.* and *Varboncoeur A. P.*
The presence and biologic activity of cementumbound endotoxins. J. Periodontol., 1974, 45: 672–675.

2. *Alexander A. G.*
The effect of subgingival scaling on gingival inflammation. J. Periodontol., 1969, 40: 717–720.

3. *Ambrose J. A.* and *Detamore R. J.*
Correlation of histologic and clinical findings in periodontal treatment: effect of scaling on reduction in gingival inflammation prior to surgery. J. Periodontol., 1960, 31: 238.

4. *Arno A., Waerhaug J., Lövdal A.* and *Schei O.*
Incidence of gingivitis as related to sex, occupation, tobacco consumption, toothbrushing and age. Oral Surg., 1958, 11: 587–589.

5. *Axelsson P.* and *Lindhe J.*
Effect of controlled oral hygiene procedures on caries and periodontal disease in adults. Results after 6 years. J. Clin. Periodontol., 1981, 8: 239–248.

6. *Axelsson P.* and *Lindhe J.*
The significance of maintenance care in the treatment of periodontal disease. J. Clin. Periodontol., 1981, 8: 281–294.

7. *Badersten A., Nilvéus R.* and *Egelberg J.*
Effect of non-surgical periodontal therapy. I. Moderately advanced periodontitis. J. Clin. Periodontol., 1981, 8: 57–72.

8. *Badersten A., Nilvéus R.* and *Egelberg J.*
Effect of nonsurgical periodontal therapy II. Severely advanced periodontitis. J. Clin. Periodontol., 1984, 11: 63–76.

9. *Badersten A., Nilvéus R.* and *Egelberg J.*
Effect of nonsurgical periodontal therapy III. Single versus repeated instrumentations. J. Clin. Periodontol., 1984, 11: 114–124.

10. *Barrington E. P.*
An overview of periodontal surgical procedures. J. Periodontol., 1981, 52: 518–528.

11. *Bower R. C.*
Furcation morphology relative to periodontal treatment. J. Periodontol., 1979, 50: 23–27.

12. *Cumming B. R.* and *Löe H.*
Consistency of plaque distribution in individuals without special home care instruction. J. Periodontal Res., 1973, 8: 94–100.

13. *Helldén L. B., Listgarten M. A.* and *Lindhe J.*
The effect of tetracycline and/or scaling on human periodontal disease. J. Clin. Periodontol., 1979, 6: 222–230.

14. *Hill R. W., Ramfjord S. P., Morrison E. C., Appleberry E. A., Caffesse R. G., Kerry G. J.* and *Nissle R. R.*
Four types of periodontal treatment compared over two years. J. Periodontol., 1981, 52: 655–622.

15. *Hughes T. P.* and *Caffesse R. G.*
Gingival changes following scaling, root planing and oral hygiene: a biometric evaluation. J. Periodontol., 1978, 49: 245–252.

16. *Jones S. J., Lozdan J.* and *Boyde A.*
Tooth surface treated in situ with periodontal instruments. Scanning electron microscopic studies. Brit. Dent. J., 1972, 132: 57–63.

17. *Jones W. A.* and *O'Leary T. J.*
The effectiveness of in vivo root planing in removing bacterial endotoxins from the roots of periodontally involved teeth. J. Periodontol., 1978, 49: 337–342.

18. *Kerr N. W.*
Treatment of chronic periodontitis. 45% failure rate after 5 years. Brit. Dent. J., 1981, 150: 222–224.

19. *Knowles J. W., Burgett F. G., Nissle R. R., Shick R. A., Morrison E. C.* and *Ramfjord S. P.*
Results of periodontal treatment related to pocket depth and attachment level. Eight years. J. Periodontol., 1979, 50: 225–233.

20. *Knowles J., Burgett F., Morrison E., Nissle R.* and *Ramfjord S. P.*
Comparison of results following three modalities of periodontal therapy related to tooth type and initial pocket depth. J. Clin. Periodontol., 1980, 7: 32–47.

21. *Lang N. P., Cumming B. R.* and *Löe H.*
Plaque development as it relates to toothbrushing frequency and gingival health. J. Periodontol., 1973, 44: 396–405.

22. *Lang N. P.*
Die Vorbehandlung in der Parodontaltherapie. Dtsch. Zahnärztl. Z., 1978, 33: 3–7.

23. *Lang N. P., Morrison E. C., Löe H.* and *Ramfjord S. P.*
Longitudinal therapeutic effects on the periodontal attachment level and pocket depth in beagle dogs. I. Clinical findings. J. Periodontal Res., 1979, 14: 418–427.

24. *Lindhe J., Hamp S. E.* and *Löe H.*
Plaque induced periodontal disease in beagle dogs – a 4-year clinical, roentgenographical and

histometric study. J. Periodontal Res., 1975, 10: 243–255.

25. *Lindhe J., Westfelt E., Nyman S., Socransky S. S., Heijl L.* and *Bratthall, G.*
Healing following surgical/nonsurgical treatment of periodontal disease. A clinical study. J. Clin. Periodontol., 1982. 9: 115–128.

26. *Lindhe J., Socransky S. S., Nyman S., Haffajee A* and *Westfelt E.*
Critical probing depths in periodontal therapy. J. Clin. Periodontol., 1982, 9: 323–336.

27. *Listgarten M. A., Lindhe J.* and *Helldén L.*
Effect of tetracycline and/or scaling on human periodontal disease. Clinical microbiological and histological observations. J. Clin. Periodontol., 1978, 5: 246–271.

28. *Löe H., Theilade E.* and *Jensen S. B.*
Experimental gingivitis in man. J. Periodontol., 1965, 36: 177–187.

29. *Lövdal A., Arno A., Schei O.* and *Waerhaug J.*
Combined effect of subgingival scaling and controlled oral hygiene on the incidence of gingivitis. Acta Odontol. Scand., 1961, 19: 537–555.

30. *Morrison E. C., Lang N. P., Löe H.* and *Ramfjord S. P.*
Effects of repeated scaling and root planing and/or controlled oral hygiene on the periodontal attachment level and pocket depth in beagle dogs. I. Clinical findings. J. Periodontal Res., 1979, 14: 428–437.

31. *Morrison E. C., Ramfjord S. P.* and *Hill R. W.*
Shortterm effects of initial nonsurgical periodontal treatment (hygiene phase). J. Clin. Periodontol, 1980, 7: 199–211.

32. *Mousquès T., Listgarten M. A.* and *Phillips R. W.*
Effect of scaling and root planing on the composition of human subgingival microbial flora. J. Periodontal Res., 1980, 15: 144–151.

33. *O'Bannon J. Y. Jr.*
Gingival tissues before and after scaling the teeth. J. Periodontol., 1964, 35: 69–80.

34. *Pihlström B. L., Ortiz-Campos C.* and *McHugh R. B.*
A randomized four-year study of periodontal therapy. J. Periodontol., 1981, 52: 227–242.

35. *Rabbani G. M., Ash M. M.* and *Caffesse R. G.*
The effectiveness of subgingival scaling and root planing in calculus removal. J. Periodontol., 1981, 52: 119–123.

36. *Raeste A-M.* and *Kilpinen E.*
Clinical and radiographic long-term study of teeth with periodontal destruction treated by a modified flap operation. J. Clin. Periodontol. 1981, 8: 415–423.

37. *Ramfjord S. P., Nissle R. R., Shick R. A.* and *Cooper H.*
Subgingival curettage versus surgical elimination of periodontal pockets. J. Periodontol., 1968, 39: 167–175.

38. *Ramfjord S. P., Knowles J. W., Nissle R. R., Shick R. A.* and *Burgett F. G.*
Longitudinal study of periodontal therapy. J. Periodontol., 1973, 44: 66–77.

39. *Ramfjord S. P.* and *Nissle R. R.*
The modified Widman flap. J. Periodontol., 1974, 45: 601–608.

40. *Ramfjord S. P., Knowles J. W., Nissle R. R., Burgett F. G.* and *Shick R. A.*
Results following three modalities of periodontal therapy. J. Periodontol., 1975, 46: 522–526.

41. *Ramfjord S. P.*
Present status of the modified Widman flap procedure. J. Periodontol., 1977, 48: 558–565.

42. *Ramfjord S. P.*
Surgical pocket therapy. Int. Dent. J., 1977, 27: 263–269.

43. *Ramfjord S. P., Knowles J. W., Morrison E. C., Burgett F. G.* and *Nissle R. R.*
Results of periodontal therapy related to tooth type. J. Periodontol., 1980, 51: 270–273.

44. *Rateitschak K. H.*
The therapeutic effect of local treatment on periodontal disease assessed upon evaluation of different diagnostic criteria. I. Changes in gingival inflammation. J. Periodontol., 1964, 35: 155–159.

45. *Riggs J. M.*
Pyorrhea alveolaris. Dental Cosmos, 1882, 24: 524–527.

46. *Robertson P. B.*
Indications, selection and limitations of surgical periodontal therapy. Int. Dent. J., 1983, 33: 137–146.

47. *Rosling B., Nyman S.* and *Lindhe J.*
The effect of systemic plaque control on bone regeneration in infrabony pockets. J. Clin. Periodontol., 1976, 3: 38–53.

48. *Rosling B., Nyman S., Lindhe J.* and *Jern B.*
The healing potential of the periodontal tissues following different techniques of periodontal surgery in plaque-free dentitions. A 2-year clinical study. J. Clin. Periodontol., 1976, 3: 233–250.

49. *Rosling B., Nyman S.* and *Lindhe J.*
Longitudinal study of surgical treatment of peri-odontal disease. Results after 6 years. J. Dent. Res., 1981, 60A: 644.

50. *Schaffer E. M.*
Histological results of root curettage of human teeth. J. Periodontol., 1956, 27: 296–300.

51. *Slots J., Mashimo P., Levine M. J.* and *Genco R. J.*
Periodontal therapy in humans. I. Microbiological and clinical effects of a single course of peri-odontal scaling and root planing and of adjunc-tive tetracycline therapy. J. Periodontol., 1979, 50: 495–509.

52. *Smith D. H., Ammons W. F.* and *Van Belle G. A.*
Longitudinal study of periodontal status compar-ing osseous recontouring with flap curettage. I. Results after 6 months. J. Periodontol., 1980, 51: 367–375.

53. *Syed S. A., Morrison E. C.* and *Lang N. P.*
Effects of repeated scaling and root planing and/or controlled oral hygiene on the periodontal attachment level and pocket depth in beagle dogs. II. Bacteriological findings. J. Periodontal Res., 1982, 17: 219–225.

54. *Stone S., Ramfjord S. P.* and *Waldron J.*
Scaling and gingival curettage. A radio-autogra-phic study. J. Periodontol., 1966, 37: 415–430.

55. *Tagge D. L., O'Leary T. J.* and *El-Kafrawy A. H.*
The clinical and histological response of peri-odontal pockets to root planing and oral hygiene. J. Periodontol., 1975, 46: 527–534.

56. *Waerhaug J.*
Microscopic demonstration of tissue reaction in-cident to removal of subgingival calculus. J. Peri-odontol., 1955, 26: 26–29.

57. *Waerhaug J.*
Effect of rough surfaces upon gingival tissues. J. Dent. Res., 1956, 35: 323–325.

58. *Waerhaug J.*
A method for evaluation of periodontal problems on extracted teeth. J. Clin. Periodontol., 1975, 2: 160–168.

59. *Waite I. M.*
A comparison between conventional gingivecto-my and a nonsurgical regime in the treatment of periodontitis. J. Clin. Periodontol., 1976, 3: 173–185.

60. *Yukna R. A.*
Longitudinal evaluation of the excisional new at-tachment procedure in humans. J. Periodontol., 1978, 49: 142–144.

61. *Yukna R. A.* and *Williams R. A.*
Five year evaluation of the excisional new attach-ment procedure. J. Periodontol., 1980, 51: 382–385.

62. *Zamet J. S.*
A comparative clinical study of three periodontal surgical techniques. J. Clin. Periodontol., 1975, 2: 87–97.

Group work

Preamble to Group Work

David E. Barmes

I have been asked to review the objectives of this Workshop and the actual work-papers, and to suggest questions for the Workshop to answer. However, I wish to start prior to the objectives by referring to the 1979 Workshop in Dublin. It was an excellent meeting and from it emerged a very useful report. I believe this follow-up Workshop to be extremely important and I want to explain why I feel that way by referring to the quotation from the 1979 Workshop which we received in our meeting papers. Let us consider the main operative sentences or phrases one by one:

1. 'Periodontal disease is a major public health problem'. – Is it? It is clearly a major *dental* public health problem, and it may have important economic aspects in terms of treatment sought and obtained that might have been avoided by prevention. However, this Workshop needs to think carefully about the criteria for declaring that periodontal disease is a *major* public health problem.
2. 'It causes much personal distress . . .' – Yes, but so do many diseases and conditions which are trivial in relation to the sum total of human suffering.
3. '. . . leads to tooth loss . . .' – Sometimes, without doubt, but what is the real impact of periodontal disease on *total* tooth loss? It may be less than we have recently assumed.

4. 'It is preventable . . .' – Yes, at least gingivitis and calculus are and mainly by self-help in terms of improved oral hygiene behaviour.
5. '. . . treatable by currently available methods.' – I trust that is correct, but can we clearly define which conditions can be successfully treated and by which methods?

There are important challenges to this Workshop, just in those five statements and the questions they pose. Moreover, Europe is not just one of many regions in the world. It has a special responsibility because the world looks to it for guidance and often follows its lead, even when relevance for transfer of technology, methodology or system does not exist.

You are mostly experts, naturally enthusiastic about your chosen specialty, but I plead with you to keep things in perspective in making decisions and recommendations which will affect the health of people, not only in relation to oral health but also, for better or worse, more generally according to the resources you use or misuse in dealing with oral health.

Objectives

The actual objectives and their details are given under six main headings. They are excellent for the purpose of this Workshop, my main misgiving being whether they could be achieved in 2½ days. I shall not dwell on them, as relevant comments will emerge from my review of workpapers and from the questions which I will suggest at the end of this preamble. I shall only emphasize the point that all the Workshop objectives are interdependent, as are the four group topics. Thus, there will be the need for repeated exchange between the groups if we are to avoid conflict and irrelevancy in our work.

Workpapers

Once more, excellence is the term with which I would refer to this set of papers. I am most impressed by the fact that they concentrate on broad concepts of what might best improve people's health rather than on the gadgetry and sophisticated procedures which so often consume our most productive moments. My review will follow the *Objective and Working Group* sequence.

Identification of the Problem

I would highlight the following points;

1. Up to very recently, population data on periodontal disease has been inadequate, irrelevant to specific needs for services and only crudely comparable, leaving room for considerable doubt.
2. With a few exceptions, we can be sure of only one broad population contrast, namely that communities in developing countries have higher scores on the various indices used than those in industrialized countries, especially where the priority for oral health, either stated or *de facto*, has been relatively high.
3. That contrast is mainly at the level of gingivitis and calculus, rather than at the more intense levels of the disease.

4. I believe that gingivitis and calculus account for more than 80% of all periodontal disease scores up to mature adulthood and that prevalence of these conditions is reducing in industrialized countries quite rapidly, though that latter opinion awaits sound evidence.
5. There is evidence that socioeconomic status is an important factor in periodontal disease experience, presumably because of different oral hygiene regimes but also, perhaps, due to different growth and development backgrounds. This contrast appears to cross all borders and needs to be better defined.
6. Our knowledge of how much tooth loss is actually caused by periodontal disease at various ages is sadly deficient.
7. We need much more data on periodontal disease, regularly, and I believe that the Community Periodontal Index of Treatment Needs (CPITN), plus tooth loss data, will be the answer to that need.
8. Comparative studies sometimes report clinically significant differences that are not statistically significant and very many report statistically significant differences which are clinically trivial. There is a need to combine these two types of significance.

Analysis of Existing Services

Central to this issue are the factors of primary health care, community and multisectoral involvement, self-care, high technology and specialization, and the balance between prevention and cure. At this stage it is appropriate for me to refer to some of the aspects of WHO's goal of *Health for All by the Year 2000*.
The orientation of services should be to promote health while developing self suffi-

ciency in communities and by progressively reducing the need for intervention.

Every shining new health facility represents failure *not* success, as the brave words at the gala opening ceremonies might suggest. Let us also note that the same applies to every health school that opens or even continues. Even to this day, one hears prevention expressed in terms of greater frequency of visits to health facilities as if this development is a virtue, whereas such visiting needs should be regarded as a necessary evil to be eliminated as quickly as possible.

Existing periodontal disease treatment services have been criticized in several of the papers for their orientation towards treatment, high technology and specialization, leading to fragmentation of care. The lack of awareness of the ways in which communities can be led to better health behaviour is also seen as a deficiency, as is the tendency to be dentist-oriented. Financing on a fee per item of service basis is indicated as a pressure towards intervention rather than prevention.

On the other hand, the description of services provided under the social security system in the Federal Republic of Germany (FRG) gives us an excellent example of a highly sophisticated system which has undeniable advantages at individual, community and health worker level. However, combined with those advantages are many of the disadvantages expressed in the papers about existing services. Also from the FRG comes a report of spectacular success in preventing oral diseases in young children, a feature of the service being the involvement of parents.

Perhaps there is some way of relating to existing structures so that their advantages can be retained and their disadvantages replaced by more desirable and effective approaches.

Because I believe that the need for change is so great in the whole oral health sector that dentistry may no longer be recognizable as an entity after 3 or 4 more decades, I want to take issue with a point made in one of the papers and to salute the profession in all its forms for its achievements; not the least being that it may engineer, as is right and proper, its own demise. That statement reads '. . . of all health services, dental services are one of the least equitably distributed'.

If we define services only as the clinical intervention type of activity, that statement may well be true, though the same limitation would need to be applied to other health sectors. However, if one includes preventive efforts, as I do, in the definition of services, then the dental profession where it is most developed and, by the way, most liberal, has achieved perhaps the most spectacular change ever achieved in the prevalence of a ubiquitous disease – dental caries. I believe it is on the way to doing the same with periodontal disease. Further, I believe that this salutation is deserved by the profession, even though much of the change may have been achieved by water or other engineers, cosmetic or pharmaceutical companies or other nonclinical agents or agencies, as it has been the influence of the profession, surely, that has set all this change in motion?

Goals

Again, I would like to commence with a *Health for All* type of statement. Our overall goal, in whatever health area we work, is to develop health behaviour and status in communities to the extent that there is no need to seek health services. In other words, this is the concept *Zero*. That is not going to happen overnight, or even by the year 2000, but every endeavour should have that goal fully in view and this Workshop should be able to take an important leadership step in that direction.

Many of the papers have given excellent suggestions for establishment of measurable goals on the way to permanent, self-maintained periodontal health. Some of the ingredients are:

1. The concept of what needs to be achieved in terms of acceptable levels of some of the clinical signs by which we measure the problem, including the number and configuration of teeth which meet the criteria of acceptability.
2. The need to stratify our goals by age and social order, and to build those goals into a national strategy for coordinated prevention.
3. The essential role of communities in decision-making and action in relation to national goals.
4. Definition of what can be achieved by various preventive and treatment programmes in relation to all levels of periodontal disease.
5. Acceptance of a monitoring system to evaluate goal achievement.

Nevertheless, there still appears some goal approaches in the papers which talk of reducing this, or improving that, without quantifying how much and from what. These quantifications may need to be added to a goal, which is at first only an intention, but it should be made clear from the beginning that such a goal will not be definitive until the measurability factor has been added.

Strategies and Manpower

We have been given an excellent format for development of strategies with which to achieve our goals. Recalling the need for integration with other health sectors, and with it the need to consider what would be appropriate nonhealth, health auxiliary and health professional personnel to pursue those strategies, it is proposed that there should be a *population strategy*, a *high technology strategy* and a

secondary prevention strategy. The first of these involves education and change at many levels and the second stresses a point, so often ignored, that social as well as clinical signs should be used for assessing high risk. Of course, age is also important and we have been alerted to the possibility that quite different approaches may be necessary by socioeconomic status and ethnicity. The third pillar of this format uses the term 'secondary prevention' which, along with similar terms such as 'complementary care', is attractive in giving the preventive first message.

In our considerations, we should heed several warnings, such as the likelihood that health spending may soon undergo, or may already be experiencing, severe and prolonged (dare we say permanent) limitation, and a caution about whether to expect an increased need for periodontal care. I would like to add my own comments. Concerning the first of these warnings, I believe that the strategy which will emphasize self-reliance as the fundamental precept of *Health for All* will surely lead to more reluctance to spend on high technology in health. As for the second warning, I would be even more cautionary.

I have already spoken of my belief that the prevalence of gingivitis and calculus is rapidly reducing and that more than 80% of what we call 'periodontal disease' is manifested by those conditions. If my belief is correct, and our efforts intensify that trend, as they should, the extra teeth saved by lower caries prevalence, thereby providing more tissues at risk, will probably not even compensate for the much lower treatment needs.

Those warnings are particularly important as we think of appropriate personnel, in quality and quantity in Europe, where dental manpower surpluses have either arrived or are just about to overwhelm our best efforts to cope with the problem. How very important it is for us to clarify these questions not only for Europe's present plight, but to avoid setting developing countries on a similar unnecessary road which many are, indeed, already following.

Other features of the papers in relation to this topic are:

1. The emphasis on health education, thus '... the major thrust of activities in preventive periodontal programmes should be aimed at mass plaque control: increasing public awareness, developing planned health education, using social and educational strategies and encouraging oral cleanliness through self-care'.
2. The need to choose between several types of intervention for a given level of disease and to consider cost effectiveness, based on longitudinal studies, as we evaluate the effects of various approaches on gingivitis, loss of attachment and loss of teeth.
3. The definition of various ways of monitoring and evaluating our progress, and of screening, including adjustable indications using the CPITN system for when to provide various educative or treatment services.
4. The need for social security and public health systems to respond to the goals and strategies defined.

Questions

The burning questions, which seem to me to emerge from this review and which I would love to see this Workshop answer, are listed below, again under the four main headings used in the review.

Definition of the problem

1. Is CPITN endorsed as the basic tool for epidemiology and monitoring of periodontal treatment needs?
2. Should it be supplemented by other monitoring tools such as nonbleeding papillae (NBP), use of x-rays, measurement of bone loss and microbiological tools? If so, which?
3. What should be the essentials of national approaches to and programmes of data collection using these tools?
4. What special efforts should be made to ascertain the contribution of periodontal disease to tooth loss?
5. Can clinical significance be defined for the various indices and measurements, and used as a filter to reduce the confusion caused by reports of statistical significance for results which are clinically meaningless?
6. What is the rating of periodontal disease as a public health problem?

Analysis of existing services

1. What are the main deficiencies of existing services in Europe in regard to periodontal health?
2. What have been the main achievements of existing systems in prevention and treatment?
3. How can social security systems and public health services be modified to optimize periodontal health of the public?

Goals

1. Can the overall statement of our periodontal health goal be '... the long life maintenance of a dentition which is functional, socially acceptable and does not pose a threat to the general health of the individual'?
2. If this overall statement or something similar is acceptable, what quantitation can we give to acceptable levels, at different ages, of gingivitis, calculus, pocketing, bone loss and tooth loss, e.g. are 24 teeth prior to 45 years and 20 teeth from 45 years onwards acceptable?

3. If these quantitations are made, can they be used to indicate, again at various ages, what are the limits for various types of services?
4. What modifications of these quantitative statements, if any, need to relate to various socioeconomic status levels and work/life situations?
5. What process can be recommended for combining these measurable statements into a National Strategy for Coordinated Prevention?
6. How can community decision-making and action be built into that process?
7. How will goal achievement or failure be monitored?

Strategies and manpower

1. What steps can be taken to integrate oral health with all health activities in establishing our response to the periodontal disease problem?
2. Is it accepted that our response will be at three levels – a population strategy, a high risk strategy and a secondary prevention strategy?
3. If that three-level response is accepted, how will each of the three programmes be structured, financed and monitored? Specifically:

(a) What will be the health education approach at various levels and how will we measure its success?
(b) How will we define high risk, deal with it and monitor our achievements?
(c) What will be the structure and procedures used in our secondary prevention programme – can some presently used procedures be deleted?
4. What will be the role of social security and public health systems in these strategies?
5. What types of nonhealth, health, dental auxiliary and dental professional personnel do we need to fulfil the tasks defined by those strategies?
6. On the subject of health education, if knowledge is not enough to ensure optimal behaviour, what else is needed and does it differ for self-care and for utilization of services?
7. Is there an effective treatment to prevent bone loss by age 15 and how should it be measured?
8. What technological developments, e.g. antiplaque toothpaste, should be supported?
9. Are socioeconomic status and sex constant variables in relation to all stages of periodontal disease and, if so, is the difference due only to different levels of hygiene?

Group Reports and Recommendations

Total Population Approach

General Considerations

The group decided that the approach should be through primary prevention, by providing information through health education for all sections of the population at risk. This would involve the identification of target groups and the development of appropriate strategies for these groups.

Identification of Relevant Problems

The main difficulty identified was the lack of awareness in the public and the profession of the value of periodontal health. Scientific research during the last decade has conclusively demonstrated that periodontal health can be maintained.

Overall Goal

The overall goal should be the promotion of a good standard of self-care in the whole population in order to maintain a healthy periodontium.

The definition of a healthy periodontium would be a matter for the profession to determine. However, the definition should include reference to the level of plaque, retention factors and mild gingival inflammation that would be compatible with the absence of progressive loss of bony support and which could therefore be tolerated.

Measurable Objectives

Before measurable objectives can be defined, target groups need to be identified. These groups will depend upon local considerations and will be based upon age, social and cultural factors. In addition it will be necessary to influence leaders of opinion in the community.

Measurable objectives for each target group need to be stated. Objectives should be stated not only in terms of clinical status, but also in terms of knowledge levels, attitudes and behaviour.

There should be overall objectives for the EEC. However, in applying these objectives, due account would need to be taken of national variations.

There need to be minimum objectives for the education of the dental profession in the EEC countries.

Strategies Including Manpower

Overall strategies

There is a need for national policies for prevention by government and national organizations. These should be based upon coordinated national programmes of dental health education integrated into general education.

With regard to younger age groups, health education should be a programmed, long-term, systematic, integrated part of nursery school and school curricula. It should be distinguished from the incidental, isolated provision of health information.

There was general agreement on the need for nonhealth personnel, under professional control, to implement field programmes.

Education of dentists

Training in periodontology should be included in, and given proper emphasis in, the dental curriculum. This should embrace aspects of psychology and sociology and also communication skills.

Continuing education of dentists in all aspects of periodontal care is necessary.

Auxiliary personnel

The various categories of auxiliary personnel should be defined in terms of the skills and knowledge required and their functions. Basically what is necessary are persons who are competent to give dental health education.

Nonhealth professionals

There is a need for nonhealth professionals, such as teachers, to be involved in dental health education.

Assessment of Progress

Periodic evaluation of change should be made according to the same measurable criteria as were employed in the setting of objectives.

The need for research

Research should be directed towards
- improved methods of preserving periodontal health;
- interdisciplinary studies of methods of affecting behaviour change.

Summary and Recommendations

1. A shift in allocation of resources from treatment to prevention should be encouraged.
2. Policies at appropriate levels for the prevention of periodontal disease should be developed. These should be based upon coordinated programmes of dental health education integrated with general health education.
3. Training in periodontology should be included, and given proper emphasis in the dental undergraduate curriculum. This should embrace aspects of psychology and sociology and also communication skills. Furthermore, continuing education of dentists in all aspects of periodontology should be given priority.
4. Periodic evaluation of changes in disease levels, public awareness, attitudes and behaviour should be made and used for adjusting priorities.

High-Risk Approach

General Considerations

The group considered the concept of 'high-risk' and defined three possibilities. For each of these possibilities, goals were defined, measurable targets identified and a strategy considered. The group report concludes with recommendations for research. The concept of a high-risk approach to periodontal disease must be considered in conjunction with a population strategy and/or a secondary prevention approach. This is in agreement with the WHO 'primary health care concept'.

People who do not have periodontitis but who are more likely to get periodontitis than the population at large.

Examples
People with high plaque scores.
Low socioeconomic groups.
Certain ethnic groups.
There is also an intraoral variation in the levels of severity of periodontal diseases.

Overall goal
To avoid the onset of loss of attachment before 18 years of age.

Measurable targets
Percent of people with attachment loss at 18 years of age.

Strategy
Primary prevention.
Development of self-assessment and self-care programmes.
Endorse WHO concept of primary health care.
Develop screening techniques to identify high risk groups.

People who have periodontitis and who are at greater risk of more severe levels of inflammatory gingivitis and/or subsequent tooth loss than the population at large.

Examples
People with:
high plaque scores;
early attachment loss;
mental/physical handicaps, e.g. Down's Syndrome;
extensive iatrogenic factors;
blood dyscrasias;
certain altered hormonal influences.

Overall goal
To maintain a functioning dentition for life.

Measurable targets
The percentage of people
with full dentures;
who wear partial dentures;
with at least 20 teeth in function;
who claim to chew satisfactorily;
who claim to be happy with the appearance of their dentition.

243

Strategy
Establish maintenance programmes.
Develop team concepts.
Establish peer review and other forms of quality control.
Establish a biological basis for dental education.
Develop a comprehensive dental care approach in dental education.
Consider screening programmes.

People with certain systemic conditions whose general health is at risk because of the presence of periodontitis.

Examples
Patients
at risk of infective endocarditis;
with blood dyscrasias;
who undergo radiation therapy.

Overall goal
Maintenance of general health and well-being.

Measurable targets
The percentage of people whose periodontal health puts their general health at risk
The percentage of 'at-risk' patients who receive a careful dental examination

Strategy
Examine all at-risk patients.
Develop hospital dental services.
Place greater emphasis on these groups in dental education.

Recommendations

The approach in health care should be along the principles of primary health care, with its emphasis on primary prevention.

In a large part of the population it is possible to maintain a functional dentition throughout life, primarily through self-care supplemented by a limited amount of professional care. There remains, however, a certain percentage of the population who comprise the high-risk group, people who are more likely to get rapidly progressing periodontal disease leading to early tooth loss. There is a basic requirement to identify these people and give them effective care.

Research is therefore needed to:

1. Develop better prognostic indicators of people at risk of:
   (a) tooth loss;
   (b) attachment loss;
   (c) deterioration in general health related to periodontal disease.
2. Understand the natural history, pathogenesis and public health significance of periodontal disease in various populations.
3. Develop the concept of a 'functional dentition'.
4. Develop self-assessment techniques and promote self-care.
5. Investigate mechanisms for implementing preventive and therapeutic techniques in the community which have been shown to be effective in clinical trials.

Secondary Prevention Approach

Definition

Taking into consideration the WHO Technical Report 621,[1] secondary prevention is defined as the treatment of the signs and symptoms of disease of the periodontium in order to prevent their progression.

Aims

To arrest, in the longterm, progression of attachment loss, taking into account minimum anatomical requirements for aesthetic, social and functional needs, as predicted or specified for particular groups and individual cases.

Identification of Problems

1. Comparable epidemiological data are lacking concerning the prevalence of periodontal disease controlled for age and severity. In addition, more information is needed concerning the relationship between sociocultural factors and periodontal disease states. Also data is needed on the discrepancies between current knowledge, dental education and dental practice.
2. There is a need for improved training in periodontology in the education of dental professionals.
3. Since well-defined prognostic indicators are still lacking, defining treatment needs – taking into account disease levels and risk factors – remains difficult.
4. Operative dental procedures, or appliances, may increase oral hygiene problems.

Measurable Targets

To establish collaborative community wide studies on:
1. The implementation of the CPITN system in as many member states as possible, supplemented by measurements of loss of periodontal support on a periodic random sample basis.
2. The use of relevant oral hygiene aids.
3. The priority given to periodontal health by patients and professional dental workers.

The use of postgraduate and continuing education in periodontology for dental professionals.

To evaluate changes in the relative proportion of preventive care as opposed to other aspects of dentistry.

Strategies and Recommendations

1. Manpower

(a) Training in periodontology must be included through-out the curriculum for all dental professionals, involving all subject divisions within schools, and with different categories of dental workers learning together on an integrated basis.

(b) Restorative dental treatment and appliances are considered potential hazards to periodontal health. This problem should be stressed in the dental curriculum and education.

(c) Postgraduate training of dental professionals should give a high priority to periodontology.

(d) National legislations permitting the free movement of oral hygienists between the EEC countries should be encouraged.

(e) The use of experts in periodontology on an ambulant community basis to give advice and consultation for workers in the field should be developed.

2.

The inclusion of secondary prevention of periodontal disease in national health policies, and an increase in resources devoted to this purpose are encouraged. Measures of secondary prevention should be universally available with appropriate quality control and designed to correct the inbalance of resources between prevention and therapy. Experiments on capitation payment systems within this field are recommended.

3.

The institution of population screening and referral by supervised auxiliary workers are recommended; expert diagnosis would occur at the treatment level.

4.

The creation and expansion of liaison with other health and education agencies in order to increase the effectiveness of secondary prevention strategies is encouraged.

5.

Evaluation of strategies should include measurement of:

(a) Treatment need changes using the CPITN system related to baseline examination.

(b) Changes in the demand for oral hygiene aids.

(c) Changes in expenditure related to secondary prevention compared to other dental treatment.

(d) Changes in rates of tooth loss.

(e) Changes in attitudes of the public and dental workers.

(f) Changes in the use of auxillary workers and their impact in treatment situations.

The Need for Research

Field research on the impact upon maintenance care of surgical *vs* non-surgical techniques for treatment of pockets is recommended. This research should include cost benefit studies to evaluate factors that influence the maintenance of treatment results.

Once comparable results are available, a further EEC workshop should be called.

Reference

1. WHO. Epidemiology, etiology and prevention of periodontal disease. World Health Organization Technical Report Series, 1978, 621: 21, WHO, Geneva.

Treatment Types and Efficacy

The group defined nonsurgical treatment as oral hygiene instruction and reinforcement and the nonsurgical root planing of root surfaces followed by a phase of healing and evaluation.

In gingival inflammation *without* loss of connective tissue attachment, proper oral hygiene may eliminate the disease. Professional aid may not be necessary in all cases.

In gingival inflammation combined *with* loss of connective tissue attachment, nonsurgical treatment, as defined above, has been shown to be effective in eliminating inflammation, reducing probing depth and maintaining acceptable attachment levels.

In areas of inaccessability of root surfaces, surgical flaps may be needed to achieve access.

Additional activities such as deliberate removal of soft tissue pocket lining, bone recontouring and placement of implants into bony defects, as well as mucogingival surgery to increase the width of the keratinized gingiva, do not appear to provide additional benefits.

To maintain treatment results, regular maintenance care has been demonstrated to be mandatory for preventing the recurrence of the disease.

The skilful performance of both the patient and the one who delivers the treatment is essential for the efficacy of any treatment.

Plenum Discussion and Recommendations

During the plenum session, several topics and statements from the group reports were reconsidered and additional aspects were brought up.

Since votes were not taken, the following formulations should not be construed as representing unanimity. However, it is the impression of the editor that this account represents a general consensus of the workshop.

The question whether periodontal disease is a major public health problem was again raised. The plenum was divided on this issue, but there was agreement that periodontal disease constitutes a major dental health problem, and that part of this problem is that there is too little public and professional awareness of the problem. It was also agreed that maintenance of periodontal tissue support of the teeth should be a public health *goal*.

Concern was expressed in relation to the use of 'periodontal health' in goal descriptions. It was considered unrealistic (and possibly undesirable) that the public health responsibility should be to eliminate incipient gingival inflammation. Rather, it should be to *limit* the progression of gingivitis to destructive periodontal disease.

The plenum recognized a need for developing methods by which periodontal disease activity may be assessed. Such methods should be applicable on a population basis in order to identify people at risk to destructive periodontal disease.

Most of the data on longterm effects of periodontal treatment stem from clinical trials. There is a strong need to carry such investigations to the level of community tests.

Maintenance care in relation to periodontal therapy needs to be defined more precisely. Further, considerations of the role of maintenance services in dental care programmes should take into account all people not in a position to avail themselves of such services. A remedy might be to develop relative independence of professional services by a high level of self-care.

The increased control of dental caries now apparent in European countries may affect the need for periodontal treatment in opposite directions. The preservation of more teeth into higher age groups will lead to more teeth at risk to periodontal disease. Conversely, the decreased need for restorative treatment may result in less iatrogenic periodontal disease.

Methods of remuneration and quality control of dental care systems should be examined as to their relevance in the prevention and treatment of periodontal disease.

The nature of dental caries and its sequelae has made it relatively easy to convince politicians and decision-makers of the need for countermeasures. Public demand will convince politicians, but there is very little public demand in relation to periodontal disease. There is a need to develop descriptions concerning periodontal disease capable of impressing politicians. National dental organizations of the EEC countries should be invited to consider:

1. Initiatives concerning the priority and awareness of periodontal disease among their own members.
2. A convention of all dental health educators and health education agencies to consider a coordinated approach to the prevention fo periodontal disease as a major dental health problem.
3. The preparation of a detailed case for health policies that support the prevention of periodontal disease.

The subject of community dental health should be included in the dental undergraduate curriculum where this is not already the case. Measures aimed at the control of periodontal disease should be given proper weight in the teaching of community dental health.

Goals for Periodontal Health

Goals for periodontal health for European populations were formulated as set out below.
The following periodontal health goals for the populations of Europe are based on an evaluation of present conditions and an educated guess at a considerable but yet realistic improvement by the year 2000. The presently available epidemiological data are insufficient and every effort should be made to obtain reliable base line data as soon as possible.

At age 18, 90% will have acceptable gingival health to the extent that each person has at least three healthy sextants (CPI = 0) (1)

With increased oral health awareness, gingival conditions already seem to have improved in most European countries. The 18-year-olds of the year 2000 were born in 1982. It seems realistic that this new gen-

eration can be educated and motivated to reach the stated goal. Reaching the goal would require good enough oral hygiene to ensure that no more than moderate disease occurs in any of the remaining sextants.

At age 35–44, 75% will have acceptable gingival health to the extent that each person has at least three healthy sextants (CPI = 0)

The persons of this age group were from 17 to 26-years-old in 1982. They already have better oral health than did the generation of their parents. It seems realistic that this goal can be reached with concerted action. Reaching the goal would ensure that deep pocketing (CPI = 4) would occur in no more than 5% of the persons belonging to this age group.

At age 65 and over, no more than 10% should have one or more sextants with deep pockets (CPI = 4)

Large percentages of this age group are edentulous, e.g. 70% to 80% in the UK in 1978. The persons belonging to this age group in the year 2000 were 47 or over in 1982, at which age the edentulous percentage would already be very high in most European populations. Therefore, a goal expressed in terms of healthy dentitions would be of little value. That no more than 10% will have deep pockets implies that sustained efforts are needed to improve the quality of the dentitions for those who remain dentate. Indirectly, and with time, this approach will lead also to an increase in the average number of teeth retained.

Reference:

1. *Ainamo J., Barmes D., Beagrie G., Cutress T., Martin J. and Sardo-Infirri J.*
Development of the World Health Organization (WHO) Community Periodontal Index of Treatment Needs (CPITN). Int. Dent. J., 1982, 32: 281–291.

Subject Index

Quinte∫∫ential to denti∫try.....

Goldman / Shuman / Isenberg

An Atlas of the Surgical Management of Periodontal Disease

A clearer understanding of the nature and behavioral pattern of periodontal disease attained from recent research has significantly influenced current periodontal therapy. While the patient must be motivated and taught why and how to maintain cleanliness, periodontal therapy must be directed towards creating an environment allowing cleansing of the dentition.

Whereas initial therapy consists of elimination or modification of all identifiable etiologic factors, the surgical treatment is aimed at the attainment of healthy periodontal structures. Surgical treatment of periodontal problems may be either resective or reconstructive; each has definite indications and contraindications.

The purpose of this text and atlas is to present the many proven periodontal surgical techniques currently being utilized in the management of periodontal disease. Concise, sequential explanations accompany the illustrations that were carefully selected to depict classical problems, step-by-step treatment, and final results.

ISBN 0-931386-41-1
220 Pages, 403 illustrations (354 in color)

Order 1386/0411

quinte∫∫ence
book∫

Quintessence Publishing Co., Inc.
8 South Michigan Avenue, Suite 2301
Chicago, Illinois 60603